BARKLEY
DEFICITS IN EXECUTIVE FUNCTIONING SCALE
(BDEFS)

Barkley Deficits in Executive Functioning Scale (BDEFS)

Russell A. Barkley

THE GUILFORD PRESS
New York London

A Division of Guilford Publications, Inc.
www.guilford.com

Printed in the United States of America

This book is printed on acid-free paper.

For product and safety concerns within the EU, please contact *GPSR@taylorandfrancis.com*, Taylor & Francis Verlag GmbH, Kaufingerstraße 24, 80331 München, Germany.

Last digit is print number: 19 18 17 16 15 14 13 12 11 10 9

Library of Congress Cataloging-in-Publication Data

Barkley, Russell A., 1949–
Barkley deficits in executive functioning scale (BDEFS) / Russell A. Barkley.
p. cm.
Includes bibliographical references and index.
ISBN 978-1-60623-934-6 (pbk.)
1. Neuropsychological tests. 2. Higher nervous activity. I. Title.
RC386.6.N48B373 2011
616.8'0475—dc22

2010044768

In memory of my sister, Nancy Jane Barkley, with love

About the Author

Russell A. Barkley, PhD, ABPP, ABCN, before retiring in 2021, served on the faculties of the University of Massachusetts Medical Center, the Medical University of South Carolina, and Virginia Commonwealth University. Dr. Barkley has worked with children, adolescents, and families since the 1970s and is the author of numerous bestselling books for both professionals and the public, including *Taking Charge of ADHD* and *Your Defiant Child.* He has also published six assessment scales and more than 300 scientific articles and book chapters on attention-deficit/hyperactivity disorder, executive functioning, and childhood defiance. A frequent conference presenter and speaker who is widely cited in the national media, Dr. Barkley is past president of the Section on Clinical Child Psychology (the former Division 12) of the American Psychological Association (APA), and of the International Society for Research in Child and Adolescent Psychopathology. He is a recipient of awards from the American Academy of Pediatrics and the APA, among other honors. His website is *http://www.russellbarkley.org.*

Acknowledgments

This manual and the construction of the Barkley Deficits in Executive Functioning Scale (BDEFS) would not have been possible without the assistance of others during the more than 10 years it has taken to develop, scientifically evaluate, and finally publish these latest versions of the scale. I am especially grateful to my close friend and colleague of more than 20 years, Kevin R. Murphy, PhD, for his collaboration on numerous research projects we have conducted on adults with ADHD that served to inform the development of the BDEFS and its initial validation. This should explain the numerous references in this manual to our research papers on adult ADHD generally and executive functioning (EF) specifically. I am also grateful to another dear friend and colleague of more than 30 years, Mariellen Fischer, PhD, for her collaborative work with me on the longitudinal Milwaukee Study of hyperactive children followed into adulthood, also frequently referenced throughout this manual. For the most recent summary of these extensive research programs, please see *ADHD in Adults: What the Science Says* (Barkley, Murphy, & Fischer, 2008).

In addition, I wish to express my sincere appreciation to Wendy Mansfield and Sergei Rodkin of Knowledge Networks (Menlo Park, California) for their assistance with the collection of data on the sample of U.S. adults used to create the norms for the BDEFS in this manual. I further wish to acknowledge the support and encouragement of my wife of more than 40 years, Patricia Gann Barkley, throughout the research behind this rating scale and the preparation of this manual. Finally, I continue to express my deep appreciation to Kitty Moore, Seymour Weingarten, and Robert Matloff of The Guilford Press for their acceptance, support of, and assistance with the normative project behind the BDEFS and the publication of this manual.

RUSSELL A. BARKLEY, PhD

Contents

Introduction

This manual describes the developmental history, normative data, psychometric properties, and scoring and interpretation of the Barkley Deficits in Executive Functioning Scale (BDEFS), as well as its clinical use for adults ages 18–81. The Appendix to this manual contains long forms (89 items) and short forms (20 items) of the BDEFS for both self- and other-reports. There is also a brief clinical interview based on the self-report short form for use in unusual circumstances when a patient is unable to complete a rating scale. Score sheets containing tables of norms (percentiles) are provided only for the self-report versions of the BDEFS (long and short forms).

The BDEFS is the culmination of more than a decade of research and development to identify the most useful items for the assessment of deficits in executive functioning (EF) in daily life activities in adults. The BDEFS is a *theoretically based* scale developed from models of EF in the neuropsychological literature—particularly my own (Barkley, 1997a, 1997b), but also those of others (see Chapter 1). It is also an *empirically developed* scale, based on statistical analyses identifying its reliable underlying dimensions and their occurrence in an adult sample ages 18–81 years, representative of the United States (relative to 2000 U.S. Census information). Not only is the BDEFS both empirically and theoretically based, reliable, and valid, but it is also exceptionally convenient to use. That is in large part because of the publisher's willingness to provide limited permission to photocopy the scales and score sheets for use by individual purchasers in their clinical or research practices. This will save the users much delay and inconvenience associated with the continual reordering of these items, as is commonplace in the scale-publishing industry.

This manual begins with a brief introduction to the concept of EF in neuropsychology. It then describes the developmental history of the BDEFS. This is followed by information on the normative sample, factor analysis, and other information concerning the scale's reliability, validity, and clinical utility. The information available appears to be sufficient to recommend the use of the BDEFS in a variety of circumstances. These may include clinical practice settings with patients for whom concerns about EF exist; research settings where the evaluation of EF deficits is of interest; treatment trials where a measure of response to intervention in the domain of EF is needed; or industrial–organizational settings where the screening of adults for possible deficits in EF is an important objective. I hope that you, my readers, will find the BDEFS useful in evaluating EF deficits in adult daily life activities.

CHAPTER 1

Executive Functioning

Early History of the Concept

The history of the concept of EF begins long before the term "executive functions" or "EF" actually appeared in the scientific literature in the early 1970s (Stuss & Benson, 1986; Wolf & Wasserstein, 2001). The basis for the concept originated more than 150 years ago, in scientists' initial efforts to understand the functions of the frontal lobes generally and the prefrontal cortex (PFC) specifically (see Luria, 1966). Thus when the term "EF" appeared, it was inherently conflated with the functions of the prefrontal lobes and vice versa (Pribram, 1973, 1976). Eventually EF would be referred to without regard to its localization in the brain (Butterfield & Belmont, 1977), although the implied assumption was that the PFC was largely involved in its existence. Particular attention was paid to the PFC rather than to the more obvious and nonexecutive functions of the primary, secondary, and tertiary motor programming zones of the larger frontal lobes, occurring adjacent to and more anterior to the sensory–motor strip.

Over time, this conflation has at times led to a circularity of reasoning, in that the functions of the PFC are said to be EF, while EF is then defined as the functions of the PFC. It has also led to a slippage in the discourse on EF between two separate levels of analysis: the neuropsychological level, involving thought (cognition) and motor action (behavior); and the neuroanatomical level, involving the localization of functions of the neuropsychological level to specific regions of the brain and their physiological activity (Denckla, 1996). EF is not exclusively a function of the PFC, given that the PFC has various networks of connections to other cortical and subcortical zones as well as the basal ganglia, the amygdala and limbic system, and the cerebellum (Fuster, 1997; Luria, 1966; Stuss & Benson, 1986). And the PFC may well engage in certain neuropsychological functions that would not be considered to fall under the umbrella of EF, such as simple or automatic sensory–motor activities, speech, and olfactory identification. For more on the earlier history of efforts to scientifically understand the functions of the PFC, see the textbooks by Luria (1966), Fuster (1997), and Stuss and Benson (1986).

By the 1960s, Luria noted that "one of the essential results of destruction of the frontal lobes in animals is a *disturbance of the preliminary . . . syntheses underlying the regulation of complex forms of motor operations and the evaluation of the effect of their own actions, without which goal-directed, selective behavior is impossible*" (p. 224; original emphasis). Although subsequent efforts to define EF as generally involving the maintenance of goal-directed action (Pennington, 1997; Welsh & Pennington, 1988) have credited Luria, Luria credited the earlier work of Bekhterev for identifying this essential feature of PFC functioning. In his 1905–1907 text *Fundamentals of Brain Function*, Bekhterev reportedly noted that damaging the frontal lobes results in a disintegration of goal-directed behavior, viewed as the principal function of the PFC.

Over the next 30–80 years, these major functions would be attributed to the PFC: the integration and execution of goal-directed behavior; the inhibition of more automatic actions and reactions to extraneous stimuli (distractibility); the production of delayed reactions; the evaluation of one's goal-directed actions relative to the external environment, especially in novel circumstances; and the overall intentionality or purposive quality of behavior. This makes it easy to understand just how such functions became part of the later conceptualization of EF when that specific term was eventually used to describe the neuropsychology of the PFC.

Neuropsychologists and neurologists are understandably fond of citing the first and most famous clinical case of PFC injury and the insights it provided into the functions of this brain region (and later into EF deficits). This, of course, is the case of Phineas Gage, the railroad construction foreman who suffered a penetrating head wound that destroyed a large portion of his PFC. This injury led to drastic alterations of his behavior, personality, and social conduct (Harlow, 1848, 1868). Gage and other patients with PFC damage studied in these early years demonstrated a lack of initiative or drive; a curtailing of their range of interests; profound disturbances of goal-directed behavior; a loss of abstract or categorical behavior; and emotional changes, such as a proneness to irritation, emotional instability, and indifference toward their surroundings, often superimposed on depression. Impulsive actions, trivial jokes, and even euphoria were noted to arise from lesions involving the more basal aspects of the PFC.

The first actual use of the term "executive" in reference to PFC functions occurred in the 1970s and has been attributed by others (Dimond, 1980; Fuster, 1997) to Karl Pribram (1973, 1976). Pribram (1973) referred to the executive role of the frontal cortex: " . . . the frontal cortex is critically involved in implementing executive progammes where these are necessary to maintain brain organization in the face of insufficient redundancy in input processing and in the outcomes of behavior" (p. 301). It was here, then, over 100 years after the initiation of scientific interest in the functions of the PFC, that its overarching "executive" nature was declared. The PFC is the brain's executive; its functions are therefore the executive functions. It would not be long before others employed the term "EF" with regard to a set of neuropsychological functions, independently of any linkage to or evidence of damage to the PFC (Butterfield & Belmont, 1977). In time, the "frontal lobe syndrome" noted by Luria (1966) would evolve into an "executive disorder" (Fuster, 1997) or a "dysexecutive syndrome" (Baddeley, 1986; Wilson, Alderman, Burgess, Emslie, & Evans, 1996). In the last 30 years, the frequency of use of the term "EF" has increased astronomically: It has become one of the most common terms in neuropsychological journals. The definition of EF has also increased in diversity, to a point where leading experts in neuropsychology would associate as many as 33 different functions with the term by the mid-1990s (Eslinger, 1996).

Defining EF

Alas, this diversity of opinion as to the nature of EF and the functions it comprises means that no consensus-based definition of EF is currently available. This section represents an attempt merely to provide a sampling of the numerous definitions that have appeared in the literature. It is not intended to be comprehensive or exhaustive.

One early and commonly cited view of EF was that specified by Stuss and Benson (1986) in their book on the frontal lobes:

> Executive control functions, called into action in nonroutine or novel situations, provide conscious direction to the functional systems for efficient processing of information. . . . The executive function represents many of the important activities that are almost universally attributed to the frontal lobes which become active in nonroutine, novel situations that require new solutions. These behavioral characteristics have been described by many authors and include at least the following: anticipation, goal selection, preplanning (means–end establishment), monitoring, and use of feedback (if–then statements). (p. 244)

In this definition, EF has four components (anticipation, goal selection, preplanning, and monitoring). In Stuss and Benson's (1986) model of PFC functions, these EF components are perched above two other frontal modules, which they govern: drive (encompassing drive, motivation, and will) and sequencing (encompassing sequence, set, and integration). In this model, drive and sequencing are not components of EF; they are brain functions governed by EF. "Drive" refers to basic appetitive states that are basic energizing forces. "Motivation" is conceived as being more mental/intellectual control of drive states. And "will" is undefined, but is implied to be an even higher state that governs motivation. But all are seen as governed by the executive system.

The second of these modules (sequencing) is said to be involved in organizing and maintaining bits of information into meaningful sequences, such as in the temporal integration and sequencing of behavior. Stuss and Benson cited Fuster's (1980) work in support of the existence of this module. Fuster argued that three subordinate functions are needed to organize and integrate behavior across time: anticipation (the prospective function), provisional memory (working memory), and control of interference (an inhibitory function). To these, Stuss and Benson added the synthetic capacity to form sets of related information, which allows the production of new, more complex information from available sequences of data. With this also goes the capacity for integrating a number of related and unrelated sets of information into novel knowledge (see Stuss & Benson, 1986, pp. 241–242).

The two subexecutive modules (drive and sequencing) govern the nonexecutive posterior/basal functional systems, such as attention, alertness, visual–spatial functions, autonomic emotional functioning, memory, sensory/perceptual functioning, language, motor functions, and cognition. Interestingly, perched above the EF level and atop all of these components is self-awareness (metacognition), believed to be the highest attribute of the frontal lobes (see Stuss & Benson, 1986, Figure 17-4 and pp. 246–247). It is viewed as separable from EF and hierarchically placed above it. From this perspective, it would appear that self-awareness is the chief executive that determines the activities of the lower-level functions, including the EF level.

One of the most popular definitions appearing in the literature on EF, particularly in research on children and on attention-deficit/hyperactivity disorder (ADHD) at all ages (Hinshaw, Carte, Fan, Jassy, & Owen, 2007; Martel, Nikolas, & Nigg, 2007; Rhodes, Coghill, & Matthews, 2005; Wilding, 2005; Willcutt, Doyle, Nigg, Faraone, & Pennington, 2005), is that given by Welsh and Pennington (1988):

> Executive function is defined as the ability to maintain an appropriate problem-solving set for attainment of a future goal. [It includes these components:] a) an intention to inhibit a response or to defer it to a later more appropriate time; b) a strategic plan of action sequences; and c) a mental representation of the task, including the relevant stimulus information encoded in memory and the desired future goal-state. (pp. 201–202)

Whereas many of the authors citing this definition have attributed it to Welsh and Pennington (1988), the latter authors cited Luria (1966) and, even earlier, Bianchi (1922) as the source of the definition. But, as noted above, we know that Luria (1966) credited Bekhterev with this insight as early as 1905–1907. Yet Luria, Bianchi, and Bekhterev were not defining EF, but were simply describing what they felt was an important function of the PFC—goal-directed action. Here again we see a conflation of EF with PFC functions.

In the Welsh and Pennington (1988) definition, EF comprises four elements: intentionality (goal-directedness), inhibition, planning, and working memory (the capacity for mentally representing information). Later, Roberts and Pennington (1996; see also Pennington, 1997) would reduce the model to just two components (working memory and inhibition) that interact to resolve conflicts or competition among action alternatives in goal-directed activity. Yet they, like many others before and since, acknowledged that EF is an umbrella term that "refers to a collection of related but somewhat distinct abilities such as planning, set maintenance, impulse control, working memory, and attentional control" (Roberts & Pennington, 1996, p. 105). They noted that the PFC also serves "a coordinative function, integrating component cognitive–perceptual processes across time and space" (p. 105). They stated that these may be reduced to a smaller set of core PFC processes, those being "the ability to maintain and manipulate short-term information needed for generating upcoming action (*working memory*) and the ability to inhibit inappropriate action" (p. 105). Pennington, Bennetto, McAleer, and Roberts (1996) further qualified the Welsh and Pennington definition above by saying that any definition of EF "is provisional and general" (p. 327). They also noted that some components of EF may involve non-PFC regions, whereas some PFC functions are not considered to be executive in nature. They offered no guidance as to just what essential feature would make a function executive or not, however.

A quite different approach to defining EF was taken by Lezak (1995) in her comprehensive review of neuropsychological assessment. To her,

> The executive functions consist of those capacities that enable a person to engage successfully in independent, purposive, self-serving behavior. They differ from cognitive functions in a number of ways. Questions about executive functions ask *how* and *whether* a person goes about doing something (e.g., Will you do it and if so, how?); questions about cognitive functions are generally phrased in terms of *what* or *how much* (e.g., How much do you know? What can you do?). (p. 42)

Refreshing here is the emphasis on the social importance of EF—the notion that EF is not just goal-directed or purposive in quality (as others have also emphasized), but that it is essential for socially independent behavior, and that such behavior promotes one's self-interests. Lezak went on to say:

> The executive functions can be conceptualized as having four components: (1) volition; (2) planning; (3) purposive action; and (4) effective performance. Each involves a distinctive set of activity-related behaviors. All are necessary for appropriate, socially responsible, and effectively self-serving adult conduct. Moreover, it is rare to find a patient with impaired capacity for self-direction and self-regulation who has defects in just one of these aspects of executive functioning. Rather, defective executive behavior typically involves a cluster of deficiencies of which one or two may be especially prominent. (p. 650)

The term "volition" here refers to a conscious choice of actions that are intentional or purposive in nature, and are therefore being guided by a conscious formulation of both a current and a desired future state of the individual, as well as of the goal being pursued to satisfy this desired future state. In other words, there is a willful intentionality to EF-guided behavior; it also requires the conscious generation of those motivational/emotional states that will be needed to initiate and sustain the future-directed action. Hence there is a strong motivational element in EF as Lezak defined it, and not just a cold cognitive element. Stuss and Benson (1986) and Fuster (1997) also noted this essential motivational aspect of EF. Lezak further noted that effective performance requires a capacity for self-awareness, and hence self-monitoring of that ongoing performance against the goal to be attained. That self-awareness includes not just awareness of one's physical status, but of the environmental and situational context in which one exists, and the social nature of most such contexts (self-consciousness of others).

Important for the purposes of the present manual is Lezak's (1995) emphasizing that many of the capacities involved in planning specifically, and executive functioning more generally (such as volition, choice, intentionality, self-motivation, and self-awareness), are difficult to examine by testing alone. She asserted that information about them is more likely to be derived from the person's history, the clinical observations of the individual across the period of examination, the reports of others who know the person well, and the archival records available for making an indirect ascertainment of deficits.

More recently, in connection with their own development of a rating scale for assessing executive functioning in children (and later adults), Gioia, Isquith, Guy, and Kenworthy (2000) wrote:

> The executive functions are a collection of processes that are responsible for guiding, directing, and managing cognitive, emotional, and behavioral functions, particularly during active, novel problem solving. The term *executive function* represents an umbrella construct that includes a collection of inter-related functions that are responsible for purposeful, goal-directed, problem-solving behavior. (p. 1)

The definition of EF has also been approached from an information-processing perspective. Typical of that perspective is the work of Borkowski and Burke (1996) and other investigators in this field whose work they summarized. Borkowski and Burke described EF as a set of three components directed at problem solving: task analysis (essentially defining the problem), strategy selection and revision, and strategy monitoring. Those authors also cited a different information-processing model developed by Butterfield and Albertson (1995), which views information processing as having three components: cognition, metacognition, and executive functioning.

> Cognition is all the knowledge and strategies that exist in long-term memory; this reservoir of information is critical to effective problem solving. The metacognitive level is aware of this lower level and contains models of the various cognitive processes as well as an understanding of how knowledge and strategies interconnect. Executive functioning coordinates these two levels of cognition by monitoring and controlling the use of the knowledge and strategies in concordance with the metacognitive level. (Borkowski & Burke, 1996, p. 241)

A similar information-processing view of EF explains it as follows:

> The umbrella concept of "executive control" encompasses those cognitive functions involved in the selection, scheduling and coordination of the computational processes responsible for perception, memory and action (Norman & Shallice, 1986; Shallice, 1994). . . . [EF enables] the maintenance of behavior on a goal set and calibration of behavior to context (Pennington & Ozonoff, 1996). (Ciairano, Visu-Petra, & Settanni, 2007, p. 335)

According to Martha Denckla (1996), "EF has become a useful shorthand phrase for a set of domain-general control processes" (p. 263). She then noted what these processes are likely to involve, such as inhibition and delay of responding, anticipatory set, preparedness to act, freedom from interference, and the ability to sequence behavioral outputs, as well as planning (p. 265). She attributed "distinctive future tense aspects of EF constructs: 'attention to the future,' 'prospective memory' ('remembering to remember'), or 'memory for the future' are some of the catchphrases employed" (p. 266). Denckla critically noted that many conceptualizations of EF begin with the unquestioned premise that it is whatever the frontal lobes do: The more functions we learn the frontal lobes do, the more will get added to EF, and vice versa. She rightly noted that the linkage of the two levels is a hypothesis, not a given. She also acknowledged a paper by Heilman (1994) presented at a scientific meeting, in which he referred to EF as the "how" and "when" of intentionality, fractionated into initiate, sustain, inhibit, and shift.

Problematic in these various definitions relying on goal-directed action as the overarching function of EF is this: They assert that various neurocognitive processes are essential for such action, yet (1) they often do not specify what those processes actually are; and (2) they do not indicate just what basis or rationale qualifies these to be considered "executive" processes while others, equally important for goal-directed action, are not so considered. What makes a neurocognitive process "executive" in nature? It cannot just be that it contributes to goal-directed action. Conscious sensory–motor actions can be considered to make such a contribution, yet walking or hand movements alone, for instance, would not seem to be what is meant here by the term "executive."

A quite different view of EF was proposed by Hayes, Gifford, and Ruckstuhl (1996), using a more behavior-analytic model and particularly the concept of rule-governed behavior (see Hayes, 1989). Their analysis of the elements often believed to constitute EF, as well as many of the tests used to assess EF, led them to conclude that EF is a special subset of rule-governed (verbally regulated) behavior. "Rule-governed" behavior is behavior that is being initiated and guided by verbalizations, whether self-directed or provided by others. Hayes and colleagues (1996) argued that EF tasks place people in situations where previously learned sources of behavioral regulation come into conflict with rules laid down by the task and/or examiner. Those task-specific rules are competing with behavior that is otherwise automatic and well practiced. Thus the typical automatic flow of behavior must be interrupted and delayed long enough for individuals to discover a new rule or select among previously learned rules that may apply in this situation. Yet interrupting a well-practiced behavior itself often requires that a rule be selected and followed that is initiating the delay in responding. And so in EF tasks individuals often have to implement a rule to inhibit their usual ongoing responding, even if it is just asking them a question about a task. They must then either select from among a set of relevant previously learned rules or generate a new one. The latter is a verbal means by which we solve problems. This view of EF appeared to gain little favor among traditional neuropsychologists, who seemed more comfortable using a cognitive-neuropsychological or information-processing view of EF than one derived from behavior analysis. Yet features of it would be incorporated into my own model of EF (Barkley, 1994, 1997a, 1997b) through Vygotsky's (1962) model of the internalization of self-directed speech.

In 1994, I sketched the broad outlines of a theory of EF and applied it specifically to ADHD, a relatively chronic developmental disorder of inattention, impulsivity, and hyperactivity known to be associated with various deficits in EF (Frazier, Demareem, & Youngstrom, 2004; Hervey, Epstein, & Curry, 2004; Willcutt et al., 2005). This "hybrid" theory was subsequently further developed (Barkley, 1997b) and eventually published in a book (1997b; see also Barkley, 2001). Unique to this theory of EF is that it specifies (1) that EF is self-regulation directed toward the future; (2) that self-regulation is a set of self-directed actions (often private, but not necessarily so) used by the individual to change his or her subsequent behavior so as to alter the likelihood of some future outcome (attain some goal); and (3) that there appear to be at least five of these self-directed (executive) activities. Each executive (self-directed) activity arises in the same manner as the self-direction and internalization of speech described by Vygotsky (1962). In short, each component of EF is a type of self-regulation (self-directed action intended to alter a later consequence, such as achieving a goal). Five such self-regulatory actions are elaborated in this theory, each of which is a conscious, voluntary, effortful action:

1. *Self-inhibition.* This represents (a) the capacity to suppress or otherwise disrupt or prevent the execution of a prepotent or dominant response to an event (the response that has been previously associated with reinforcement or has the highest likelihood of being performed under ordinary circumstances); (b) the capacity to interrupt an ongoing sequence of behavior toward a goal if it is proving to be ineffective; and (c) the capacity to protect the self-directed actions that will subsequently occur, and the goal-directed actions they are guiding, from interference by external and internal goal-irrelevant events.

2. *Self-directed sensory–motor action.* This is an alternative means of defining nonverbal working memory and refers to the use of self-directed visual imagery, along with the private rehearsal of visual–motor actions it permits. Although this consists largely of visual imagery, or the "mind's eye," it also consists of the other senses, such as private rehearing, retasting, resmelling, and refeeling (kinesthetic–proprioceptive experience). In totality, this component of EF provides for the conscious, willful reexperiencing of past events—a metaphorical Cartesian theater of the mind. Yet it also includes the capacity for practicing or reperforming sensory–motor actions privately to oneself, for a form of mental behavioral simulation.

3. *Self-directed private speech.* This is the alternative explanation for the verbal working memory system to that offered by information-processing models and traditional cognitive models of EF, such as Baddeley's (1986) phonological loop in his model of working memory. It is largely based on Vygotsky's (1962) theory of the internalization of speech to form the "mind's voice." Individuals talk to themselves to permit private rehearsal of utterances, as well as self-directed instructions, self-questioning, and other means by which language can be used for self-regulation and problem solving.

4. *Self-directed emotion/motivation.* This component of EF is believed to arise from the combination of the first three, in which the individual learns to use inhibition, private imagery (and private sensing more generally), and private speech to initially inhibit strong emotions and then to down-regulate or otherwise moderate them. The person then employs these other components to replace the initial strong emotion with alternate emotional responses more consistent with social demands and the individual's goals and longer-term welfare. Because emotions are motivational states, the fourth component of EF also provides for the capacity for

self-motivation—the drive states needed to initiate and sustain action toward the future.

5. *Self-directed play (reconstitution).* The fifth component of EF is an alternative to the planning, problem-solving, and inventive or generativity/fluency components noted in other views of EF. It is hypothesized to be founded on the development of play and is seen as essentially a two-step activity. The first is "analysis," or taking apart features of the environment and one's own prior behavior toward it. This is followed by "synthesis," or the regrouping of components of the environment and behavioral structures into novel combinations. These novel combinations can then be tested against a criterion, such as a problem or goal, for their likely effectiveness in overcoming obstacles to goal attainment. Although this begins as observable manual play, it progresses like the other EF components to being turned on the self and internalized as a form of private mental play. This permits both the manipulation of mentally represented information about the environment and about prior behavioral structures, so as to yield new combinations that can serve as options for goal-directed problem solving. It is possible that this component can be subdivided into both nonverbal and verbal modules that provide for fluency and generativity in each of these forms of behavior. Nonverbal, verbal, and action fluencies are believed to arise from this component of EF.

Unique to this view of EF is that it operationally defines the term (self-regulation across time toward the future), specifies its five component functions (inhibition, sensory–motor action, private speech, emotion/motivation, and play), and states why they are executive in nature (they are self-directed actions that alter future consequences). EF is thus a self-directed set of actions intended to alter a delayed (future) outcome (attain a goal, for instance). Actions that are not self-directed, including any being used to attain the goal, are not considered executive in nature. The self-directed actions that are guiding those other activities are executive.

Common Attributes in the Definitions of EF

Some broad principles involved in the concept of EF can be discerned across the history of its development:

- The vast majority of definitions emphasize the *goal-directedness* of EF. The concept therefore includes a future orientation, purposive quality, or intentionality of action.
- Some emphasize the essential element of foresight—*a sense of the future.* "Man is the animal that binds across time, binding the present to the future," as Fuster (1997) noted in his emphasis on the cross-temporal organization of behavior.
- Unspoken in most definitions of EF, though inherent in its goal-directed nature, is *a conscious awareness or sense of time, timing, and timeliness.* It is the temporal foreperiod over which events, actions, and consequences are being consciously bound together and evaluated, and decisions are being made about what is to be

desired (the goal one eventually wants to attain). It undoubtedly varies across individuals and contributes to human variation in time preference or reward discounting—the extent to which individuals decrease the value of a delayed relative to an immediate reward as a function of the time lag or delay interval (Green, Fry, & Myerson, 1994; Green, Myerson, Lichtman, Rosen, & Fry, 1996). It is a critical factor in some theories of economics and of human decision making in social exchange (Mises, 1948/1990).

- To contemplate and select from among various courses of action that may be relevant to attaining a future goal, one must consciously consider one's experience—what one has done previously in similar situations, how well it succeeded then, and how it may be applicable to the present situation and the desired goal. This is the retrospective function, or *hindsight.*

- Typically inchoate as well in most of these definitions concerns another capacity that is inherent in goal-directed action and the foresight needed to conceive of it; this is *self-awareness.* Every goal represents a want, a desire, a value, or more generally a change in a person's current state of wants and needs (a reduction in dissatisfaction, an increase in well-being or satisfaction). This represents a conflict between the current state of the individual (what he or she feels now) and what the individual wants that state to be. The conflict is, by definition, a problem for the individual. To be able to address such conflicts in state, the individual must be aware of them—that is, must be *self-conscious* of these current and future inner states.

- To conceive of a future state for oneself (hypothetical though it may be), which is to employ foresight, the individual must cease responding to the present (the now). Attention must be shifted away from the moment and toward the self and the mentally contemplated future—the goal. This requires *inhibition—especially the inhibiting of prepotent responses.*

- Many authors have noted that goal-directed action requires a set of neurocognitive processes most often identified as follows:
    - *Working memory.* Holding information in mind, such as goals and subgoals, and the means to attain them—the plan.
    - *Planning.* Mapping out the tactics and strategies (the nested sets of actions or means needed to attain the goal and any subgoals), and then constructing the cross-temporal behavioral structures and their hierarchy that will bridge the time delay and attain the ultimate goal, which of course must be held in mind.
    - *Problem solving.* The means of generating multiple possible alternative actions that may be needed when goal-directed actions (initial plans) are thwarted or unsuccessful and the plan must be revised. It may even be needed to construct the initial plan to begin with because, as noted above, goal-directed action arises when there is a conflict between a present state (what is) and a desired state (what is wanted). Such a conflict, by definition, is a problem. Hence problem solving may be invoked at the very start of creating goal-directed action. The problem-solving capacity provides for mentally testing or simulating those options for their likely success (consequences)—their ability to achieve the goal. This probably involves the capacity to manipulate

the contents of working memory or what is being held in mind. This is predominantly a process of action fluency (Piatt, Fields, Paolo, & Troster, 1999) rather than object-naming fluency. In short, the individual can conceive of various ways of doing something, and can select the one most likely to attain the goal, given his or her experience.

- *Self-monitoring.* An ongoing self-supervisory comparative feedback process that judges the adequacy of the individual's ongoing actions and their consequences (especially errors that may signal a failure of the plan) against the internally represented plan and its goal. We may infer that this capacity includes within it the capacity to *shift* (or stop and change) the ongoing stream of behavior as a consequence of this evaluative activity, reflecting as it does *a sensitivity to error* (ineffectiveness of the original plan).
- *Interference control.* A sustained inhibitory capacity to prevent interference from and responses to goal-irrelevant ongoing events (distractibility), both external and internal. This serves to protect the other EF activities from disruption (granting them a freedom from distraction).
- *Self-motivation.* The drive, the will, or the motivation needed to sustain self-directed actions toward a future goal. No matter how great the plan or mental map constructed to attain a goal may be, no self-powered, locomoting, acting entity is going anywhere without a source of fuel.

• All of these necessary functions or capacities for engaging in goal-directed actions are initiated by, directed toward, and for the benefit of the self and one's self-interests. Thus EF is, by definition, *self-regulation for the purposes of self-interests.* "Self-regulation" is any action directed at oneself that changes subsequent behavior so as to alter the likelihood of a future outcome (a goal) for the self (Barkley, 1997a, 1997b; Skinner, 1953). The chief executive is therefore *the self*—the conscious sense of oneself over time (past, present, and future), and so of one's needs, wants, and desires (self-interests) as one perceives them to be *over time.*

• Finally, we must acknowledge the fact that the goals toward which EF and its components are being used are largely *social goals and occur in the context of a social group.* Those social goals are being pursued often with others, sometimes against others, and nearly always in the larger context of others. That is the environmental niche in which EF is likely to have evolved, and the problems of this niche are the ones it probably evolved to solve (Barkley, 2001; Dimond, 1980).

I therefore define EF as *self-regulation across time for the attainment of one's goals (self-interests), often in the context of others.* EF is thus a *metaconstruct.* That is, such self-regulation across time to achieve goals, often in a social context, requires multiple, interacting mental modules or neuropsychological capacities (constructs) that all contribute to EF (the metaconstruct). Disturbances or difficulties in the effective functioning of any one module disturb EF, but in a different way from disturbances in other modules. In other words, EF, defined as self-regulation, is not one thing but involves multiple self-directed activities.

These activities or mental capacities include self-stopping (inhibition) and sustained self-protection of EF (interference control); self-awareness over time, or a conscious sense of time, past, and the future (hindsight, foresight); working memory (mentally represented information achieved by sensing to the self); self-planning and problem solving; and self-monitoring (and shifting as needed). By adulthood, many of these self-directed activities (e.g., self-awareness, visual imagery, private audition and speech, private emotion regulation, and mental play) are unobservable or very difficult to observe, and are therefore cognitive or mental in form. Others may be more public and outwardly observable (e.g., observable self-speech, writing notes to oneself, posting cues or other stimuli in one's work or living space to increase the likelihood of a later behavior, meditating to reduce a strong negative emotional state, doodling various options for solving a problem on paper, etc.). All are executive activities because all are self-directed and intended to alter a later consequence. Since a problem can be defined as a situation for which one does not have a readily available response, it is by definition a novel situation. Therefore, EF and its self-directed activities will appear to be most needed and most activated when *novelty* has been encountered.

Executive functions (self-directed activities) are not independent, but interactive and probably hierarchically organized in development. The capacity to hold information in mind (working memory), such as using visual imagery, requires that the individual inhibit responding to momentary external events and resist interference from competing sources of goal-irrelevant information (inhibition and resistance to distraction). The holding of such information in mind can be further enhanced by self-directed speech (or the phonological loop in Baddeley's model of working memory). Both of these activities (speech and imagery) may then be subjected to mental manipulation (self-directed play, or the fluency, generativity, or reconstitutive executive function) to develop multiple possible options for responding to the situation. And the emotional restraint and self-motivation that may be required to drive the goal-directed behavior toward the intended goal may be facilitated or even initiated by self-imagery and self-speech.

These, then, are the ideas that led to the construction of the initial item set for the BDEFS. The development of the BDEFS is described in the next chapter.

CHAPTER 2

Development of the BDEFS

The motivations behind the development of the BDEFS were several. One was the desire to develop a cost-effective means of conveniently capturing the numerous neuropsychological, behavioral, emotional, and motivational symptoms often attributed to deficits in EF. A second, related motivation arose from accumulating evidence that EF tests were not the most ecologically valid means for clinically evaluating EF, and were fraught with other problems that greatly limited their validity and clinical utility as putative measures of EF (Barkley & Fischer, in press; Barkley & Murphy, 2010b; Dimond, 1980; Lezak, 1995).

Problems with EF Tests

Many tests have been declared as measures of EF in the neuropsychological literature—too many to discuss in any detail here (see the meta-analyses of Frazier et al., 2004, and Hervey et al., 2004, for a lengthy list of those EF tests used just in studies of ADHD; see Lezak, Howieson, Loring, Hannay, & Fischer, 2004, for a more comprehensive review). But the virtually unquestioned premise that EF tests are the gold standard for measuring EF can be challenged on a number of grounds:

- *Many of these tests were typically not originally designed to measure EF* (see Lezak et al., 2004). Even a cursory glance at the history of EF tests shows that many were originally developed to assess other psychological functions, such as attention, memory (both verbal and visual–spatial), sequencing, abstract reasoning, and language. Others were intended to assess response inhibition, planning, and problem solving directly, without regard to these constructs' being involved in EF. And most do not assess frontal lobe (EF) functions exclusively or differentially (Dodrill, 1997). But once the umbrella term of EF was defined as including these constructs, or once it might be shown that deficits on these tests were apparently associated with injuries to the PFC, the tests were conscripted into being EF tests without regard to whether they actually were sampling the conceptual domain or construct of EF.

- *There is no consensus-based definition of EF that can serve as the standard for determining the construct or even face validity of most EF tests.* EF is quite ambiguously defined (see Chapter 1); researchers disagree on the precise meaning of the term (Castellanos, Sonuga-Barke, Milham, & Tannock, 2006; Willcutt et al., 2005). Instead, reviews of the research seem to focus more on listing the constructs thought to be subsumed under the term and the tests believed to evaluate those constructs, such as response inhibition, resistance to distraction, working memory, planning and problem solving, and set shifting (Boonstra, Oosterlaan, Sergeant, & Buitelaar, 2005; Frazier et al., 2004; Hervey et al., 2004; Willcutt et al., 2005).

- *If EF involves the cross-temporal organization and maintenance of behavior directed toward goals, as many seem to believe, it is not immediately apparent how traditional tests of EF using such small ascertainment windows to sample behavior in the clinic (typically 5–30 minutes per test) are sampling the cross-temporal nature of EF implied by these definitions.* Or if they do so, it is only for exceptionally short temporal durations relative to the hours, days, and weeks over which adults sustain their goal-directed activities. This incredibly brief ascertainment window surely must make it difficult if not impossible for EF tests alone to capture the lengthy cross-temporal structures of normal human action. This problem of grossly limited temporal ascertainment by tests alone would ensure that they are weakly related or unrelated to measures of EF taken in naturalistic settings, as by observations over days or by ratings over weeks and months. In contrast, ratings of EF in daily life ascertain behavior across considerably longer periods of time (weeks to months) and therefore serve better than EF tests may do as indicators of cross-temporal behavioral organization and problem solving directed toward goals in naturalistic settings.

- *EF tests do not evaluate some of the most important features of EF.* EF tests simply do not sample many of the capacities believed to be central to the construct of EF, as commented on by some previous authors from Luria (1966) onward, and even in the earliest descriptions of PFC injuries. As noted by Lezak (1995) (see Chapter 1), these include the constructs of volition and human will; intentionality or purposiveness; self-awareness (of self, context, and others); and even aspects of planning (foresight, objectivity, choice and comparative judgment, hierarchical structuring) and plan execution (self-motivation, self-monitoring, prolonged resistance to interference by goal-irrelevant events, etc.).

- *Moreover, given the near-consensus that EF is self-regulation, it is also not obvious how current EF tests can assess self-modification for long-term self-interestedness, self-sufficiency, and social independence—also mentioned by Lezak (1995) and Eslinger (1996), among others, as inherent in the concept of EF.*

- *If EF evolved for principally social functions, such as reciprocity and social exchange, competition, cooperation, and mutualism more generally (again, see Chapter 1), the absence of such purposes and motives in traditional EF tests would further assure their limited utility in predicting EF in daily life activities and in major domains of adaptive functioning.*

• *EF tasks are not only complex but contaminated; they involve multiple cognitive processes, many of which are not considered part of EF.* Only some of those processes are supposedly reflecting the EF construct that is intended to be sampled (Anderson, 2002; Castellanos et al., 2006). A related concern is that many EF tests are often found to be significantly influenced by overall general cognitive ability or level of intelligence (Mahone et al., 2002; Riccio, Hall, Morgan, Hynd, & Gonzalez, 1994), making their results difficult to interpret as reflecting unadulterated measures of a particular EF construct. This is likely to explain findings that statistically removing IQ from relationships between EF tests and observations and ratings of EF in natural settings often reduces any significant relationships to nonsignificant status (Mahone et al., 2002; Mangeot, Armstrong, Colvin, Yeates, & Taylor, 2002). And it may also account for the fact that some of the strongest relationships noted to date have been those between EF tests and academic achievement scores (Biederman, Petty, Fried, Black, et al., 2008; Gropper & Tannock, 2009; Thorell, 2007) or self-ratings of academic performance (Ready, Stierman, & Paulsen, 2001). Given that both academic achievement and self-rated academic performance are significantly related to IQ, and that there is a shared method (testing) when academic tests are used, this finding is not surprising. This problem of conceptual contamination is found far less often for EF rating scales whose items have been intentionally selected to directly sample the various behaviors specified in EF constructs (Barkley & Murphy, 2010b). Such scales or direct observations also have few or no significant relationships with intelligence (Alderman, Burgess, Knight, & Henman, 2003; Barkley & Murphy, 2010b), and so the issue of contamination by general cognitive ability is far less problematic for rating scales than for EF tests. Hence the conceptual or face validity of rating scales may be superior to that of EF tests, merely as a consequence of their initial construction. As noted above, many EF tests were not initially designed to measure the construct of EF.

• *Only a minority of patients experiencing frontal lobe injuries, or those with ADHD presumed to have a frontal lobe disorder, score in the impaired range on EF tests.* In contrast, the vast majority do score in this range on ratings of EF in daily life activities or in direct observations of EF performance in natural settings (Alderman et al., 2003; Barkley & Murphy, 2010b; Burgess, Alderman, Evans, Emslie, & Wilson, 1998; Kertesz, Nadkarni, Davidson, & Thomas, 2000; Mitchell & Miller, 2008; Wood & Liossi, 2006). Given the strong historical linkage of EF to PFC functioning (see Chapter 1), it is unlikely that those patients having disorders of the PFC would not likewise show impairment in EF. In regard to ADHD, however, this situation has led some to argue that ADHD is probably not a disorder of EF, given that the majority of cases have no deficits on EF tests (Boonstra et al., 2005; Jonsdottir, Bouma, Sergeant, & Scherder, 2006; Willcutt et al., 2005)—a conclusion much harder to justify logically in patients with demonstrated PFC damage.

• *EF tests have very low or no ecological validity.* That is, they correlate poorly if at all with ratings of EF in daily life activities in natural settings in adults (Alderman et al., 2003; Bogod, Mateer, & MacDonald, 2003; Burgess et al., 1998; Chaytor, Schmitter-Edgecombe, & Burr, 2006; Hummer et al., 2010; Ready et al., 2001; Wood & Liossi, 2006) or in children with frontal lobe lesions, traumatic brain injury (TBI), or other neurological or developmental disorders (Anderson, Anderson, Northam, Jacobs, & Mikiewicz, 2002; Mangeot et al., 2002; Vriezen & Pigott, 2002). This is also the case both in adults with ADHD and in children with ADHD followed to adulthood (Barkley & Fischer, in press; Barkley & Murphy, 2010a). The results of those studies usually reveal that any single EF test shares just 0–10% of its variance with EF ratings. The relationships are frequently not statistically significant. Even the best combination of EF tests shares approximately 12–20% of the variance with EF ratings or observations as reflected in these studies. Yet these two types of measurement are supposed to be measuring the same construct, EF. If IQ is statistically removed from the results, the few significant relationships found in these studies between EF tests and EF ratings may even become nonsignificant (Mangeot et al., 2002). Something is terribly amiss here if different approaches to measuring the same construct are found to be so poorly related to each other.

Additional evidence for the low ecological validity of EF tests comes from studies in which the performances of frontal-lobe-injured patients on tasks in daily life have been directly observed and correlated with EF test batteries. These studies, too, find little or no relationship between impairment in such performances and EF test results (Alderman et al., 2003; Mitchell & Miller, 2008). Here again, EF tests may account for just 9–15% of the variance or less in ratings of adaptive impairment, primarily in work activities (Ready et al., 2001; Stavro, Ettenhofer, & Nigg, 2007). In contrast, research has noted moderate relationships between EF ratings and measures of daily adaptive functioning in children with TBI and other neurological or developmental disorders (Gilotty, Kenworthy, Sirian, Black, & Wagner, 2002; Mangeot et al., 2002), as well as in adults with ADHD (Biederman, Petty, Fried, Doyle, et al., 2008), those with frontal lobe disorders (Alderman et al., 2003), and college undergraduates (Ready et al., 2001). And EF ratings substantially outpredict EF tests in the variance shared with measures of impairments in various major life activities, such as occupational functioning, educational history, driving, money management, and criminal conduct (Barkley & Fischer, in press; Barkley & Murphy, 2010a). The totality of findings to date concerning the relationship of EF tests to EF ratings and of each to impairment in daily life indicates that EF tests are largely not sampling the same constructs as are EF ratings or direct evaluations of EF in daily life (Alderman et al., 2003; Shallice & Burgess, 1991). It also provides a basis for not accepting EF tests as the primary or sole source for establishing the nature of EF deficits in various disorders.

The evidence to date indicates that if assessing how well people do in using EFs in their daily life activities is important in clinically evaluating EF, then rating scales assessing EF are superior to EF tests in doing so. Yet the very plethora of studies using tests exclusively to evaluate EF with various patient and general population samples indicates that these serious problems with EF tests have gone largely unknown, unappreciated, or ignored.

This significant failure of EF tests to relate well to EF ratings, daily life activities, or impairment in major domains of life could well indicate that the former are not assessing EF. This seems doubtful, given that many of these tests have been shown to index activities in various regions of the PFC that largely underly EF. And it is surely unlikely to be the case that EF ratings are not actually evaluating EF. After all, their item content has been drafted directly from definitions of EF and from lists of putative EF constructs in the literature, as well as from observations and clinical descriptions of patients with PFC lesions believed to manifest the "dysexecutive syndrome" (Burgess et al., 1998; Gioia et al., 2000; Kertesz et al., 2000). Moreover, as noted above, these ratings are substantially related to impairment in various daily life activities and various domains of adaptive functioning (work, education, driving, social relationships, self-sufficiency, etc.) in which EF would surely be operative.

The solution to this paradox of why EF tests and EF ratings are so poorly related lies elsewhere, most likely in the fact that EF is more hierarchically organized than models built entirely on EF tests indicate (Barkley, 2011a; Barkley & Fischer, in press; Barkley & Murphy, 2010a, 2010b). EF tests probably assess the most rudimentary, moment-to-moment, instrumental, and cognitive level of EF. But they are very poor at capturing the higher adaptive, tactical, and strategic levels of EF as they are deployed in daily adaptive functioning, human interactions, and socially cooperative and reciprocal activities that play out over much longer spans of time (days, weeks, months, and years) (Barkley, 2011a). It is at these higher, more complex, and longer-term levels that a rating scale of EF can be useful because of its use of a far longer ascertainment window for capturing summary judgments of behavior over time and because of its ability to capture EF symptoms in their important (largely social) contexts via the reports of the index person and of others who know that person well.

Also, if the purpose of evaluating EF in patients is to render some judgment as to their likelihood of experiencing impairments in major domains of life activities, then EF ratings are far superior to EF tests in doing so. On the other hand, if the purpose of the evaluation is to assess the most proximal neuropsychological EF activities related to moment-to-moment brain activity, as may be important to do in functional brain imaging studies, then EF tests may be preferable. Yet even that point is arguable in view of recent studies linking neuroimaging results to traits assessed via rating scales (Buckholtz et al., 2010). Moreover, such tests can be criticized for stripping out important social and cross-temporal elements of EF, which may reduce the validity of the task in sampling any particular component of EF or its adaptive (evolutionary) purposes.

Disadvantages of Rating Scales

In fairness, ratings of behavior, including those of EF, have their own inherent disadvantages. These problems with behavior rating scales have been discussed in detail previously (Barkley, 1987; Cairns & Green, 1979); the major points are summarized here.

- *Rating scales assume that the respondent and examiner share an understanding with regard to the nature of the item being rated and the meaning of the anchor points or potential answers being provided on the scale for responding to that item.* One source of difficulty, therefore, can be the specificity or clarity of the item to be rated, as well as the answers or anchor points being provided for the rating of the item. How well do the examiner and respondent share an understanding of the items and potential responses? The more precisely the item and its answers can be specified, the greater is the likelihood that the respondent and examiner will share an understanding of the nature of the behavior or trait to be rated and the answers to be provided.

• *The generality or ambiguity of the item being rated and the imprecision of the anchor points of the answer scaling itself, no matter how clear and specific the wording may be, can lead to problems in testing hypotheses that require far more precise measurement than the scale is likely to provide.* Such a problem arises as a consequence of the nature of a hypothesis being tested or the purpose of the assessment. To the degree that great precision in measurement is needed to fulfill that purpose or to test that hypothesis, rating scales may be a poor choice of assessment method for the construct of interest. On the other hand, there are many questions or hypotheses in psychology or purposes in clinical evaluations that do not require such a level of precision. Indeed, using excessively precise forms of measurement such as tests or direct observations of behavior is often more expensive and time-consuming than is necessary to address the issue, when a rating scale would serve just as well at far less cost and time. The potential problem of precision of measurement with a rating scale is only so when judged relative to the hypothesis being tested or intended purpose of the clinical evaluation, and not some inherent and absolute flaw of rating scales outright.

• *Various factors may influence a rater's capacity to provide an accurate report of the behavior represented in the items on the scale.* Level of intelligence, education, emotional status, range of life experiences, prior experience with similar rating scales, and a myriad of other factors have the potential to bias the rater's reports in ways that may affect the accuracy or validity of the ratings being provided. For instance, an adult's anxiety may result in an overreporting of ADHD symptoms by that adult, relative to the level reported by someone who knows the person well and is using the same scale; the same is true in EF ratings (see Chapter 7; see also Barkley, Knouse, & Murphy, in press). It is conceivable that this represents a true biasing of the rating of this person, such that it is less valid or less accurate than the rating being provided by the collateral adult. Users of rating scales clearly need to be aware of any findings from research concerning the nature of such biasing effects on the type of rating scale under consideration.

Yet it is also possible that level of anxiety actually does result in a greater degree of ADHD symptoms—or, in the present case, ratings of EF deficits in daily life—and therefore that the rater's report is not inaccurate, but simply reflecting this real impact of anxiety on EF deficits. Performance on EF tests can likewise be adversely affected by the presence of other characteristics of the examinee, and, as here, may reflect either a bias away from the true or valid level of performance or a truly adverse effect on EF performance that is not a bias at all. Obviously, far more research is needed on the issue of the extent to which other features of raters influence their ratings of EF, and whether this represents a bias or error in the rating or a true influence on the actual behavior being rated. To the extent that such biases may operate, this will contribute to measurement error, reducing the reliability and especially the validity of the rating. However, evidence to be discussed later (Chapters 6 and 7) and some already presented above indicates that despite such potential biases, rating scales may outperform EF tests in predicting adaptive functioning in daily life activities or impairment in major domains of life. Ratings therefore may still have considerable value, or, in this case, greater ecological validity, even if they offer imperfect samples of the behaviors being rated. The question here, then, in the selection of a measure is the intended purpose for which the measure is being used. Some purposes will demand the type of data that can be provided by administering an EF test or by directly observing the participant's behavior in selected settings. Other purposes can be easily fulfilled by the type of information to be gleaned from the far more cost-effective rating scale.

- *Rating scales are often criticized for using relatively vague references to frequency of behavior, such as "sometimes," "often," or "very often."* To some extent, such criticisms are quite justified if one is interested in very precise, fine-grained frequency counts of behavior, as might be gleaned from direct behavioral observations or from responses on a reaction time task. Such precise frequency counts may be necessary, in fact, to test certain psychological hypotheses. But at the level of clinical practice and judgment, and for other research purposes where such precision is often unnecessary and unduly costly and cumbersome, the more general judgments of individuals based on their own observations of themselves or others have proven to be sufficiently accurate, convenient, and inexpensive—and, more importantly, reliable, valid, and predictive—to be of great utility. Indeed, research comparing the scores derived from clinical tests, such as continuous performance tests or even driving simulators, has often found these scores to be less predictive of their respective constructs as assessed in natural settings (parent and teacher ratings of inhibition and attention, or department of motor vehicle records or reports of others about one's driving, respectively) than are ratings of an individual's test-taking behavior in that same setting completed by the examiner (Barkley, 1991; Barkley, Murphy, DuPaul, & Bush, 2002; Shelton et al., 1998). To reiterate, each approach to measurement has its place, depending on the purpose of the evaluation.

- *Critics of rating scales often charge that the ratings on a scale are more subjective than the responses of the individual to a test.* This reflects a misunderstanding of the term "subjective," I believe. The answers to rating scale items are not "subjective" and thus cannot be besmirched by this assertion alone. Thoughts, states of mind, and even privately held opinions are subjective as long as they remain in the head/mind and unobservable to others. They cannot be tested against reality for their conformance to it—that is to say, their objectivity (Popper, 1979). But once a thought is expressed publicly in any form (verbal, motor, or emotional behavior), that behavior can be observed by others and recorded, as in the case of a rating scale. The response itself, regardless of the thought it may be linked to, is an item of observable information that can be tested in various ways for its veracity (truth value) and utility. The degree to which the rating actually represents the privately held opinion of the rater may never be known. The degree to which the rating reflects the actual behavior that is to be rated, however, is a different matter and is open to empirical validation. Thus, when people report that they have considerable problems remembering things that they have been told to do, it is not of so much concern that their rating be evaluated for how well it captured their private mental state. More important is the issue of how well the rating corresponds to the level of problems these people actually have in remembering such things. The validity of the rating as an index of the problem can be investigated, whereas the validity of the rating as a reflection of a private mental state cannot. But it is rare that the latter issue is the one under consideration in the research project or clinical evaluation of a patient. It is the former issue that matters most.

To summarize, any charge of imprecision or subjectivity leveled against interviews and rating scales in an effort to disparage them without reference to further evidence concerning the purpose of the evaluation; the issue under investigation; and the evidence for the interviews' or scales' reliability, validity, and utility is baseless. The validity of relatively broad human estimates as recorded in structured interviews or rating scales concerning the relative frequency of specific behaviors is itself a form of information that can be observed, recorded, and tested, as seen in Chapter 5, for its reliability, validity and utility no differently from a response to any test. That is what matters and should be the basis on which a clinician or scientist chooses a method of measurement—not some inherent bias in favor of tests over rating scales, regardless of the issue at hand.

Whether or not the behavior of a participant is recorded by his or her circling of a response to an item on a rating scale, a button press on a device, or a verbal response recorded on some testing answer sheet is a distinction without a difference. All are forms of observable and recordable behavior, and the proof of their validity is in the evidence available about them. The widespread knee-jerk penchant of neuropsychologists to assume that a test is somehow more objective, precise, and therefore useful than a rating scale is a hypothesis; it is not a fact in the bag. The claim deserves to be subjected to testing in research and is not a fact by mere consensus of opinion or proclamation by an authority alone. So far, this assumption of the test as a gold standard of measurement has proven questionable for pursuing certain issues or purposes, such as the prediction of functioning in naturalistic settings or the determination of whether a particular disorder involves deficits in EF, such as ADHD. Clinicians, industrial/organizational psychologists, and even researchers need not apologize for using rating scales to assess certain domains of behavior and functioning, instead of some form of recording directly observed behavior or testing, if the evidence shows that those scales have merit for the intended purpose. The available evidence shows that for certain purposes rating scales are acceptable forms of measurement—in this case, of EF.

Advantages of Rating Scales

With these caveats and issues surrounding the use of rating scales for evaluating human behavior and psychological traits in mind, let us consider now a list of the advantages of rating scales for clinical and research purposes, again with the caveat that the purpose of the evaluation is the determining factor in the final analysis of the best method to assess EF. To their considerable credit, rating scales have numerous advantages (see Barkley, 1987; Cairns & Green, 1979):

- *Rating scales have the capability of gathering information from informers with many years of experience with the individuals to be rated, or with themselves if they are the subjects of the ratings.*

• *This vast experience occurs across a diversity of settings and circumstances that is nearly impossible to duplicate through any other means,* at least in any cost-effective way.

• *Rating scales permit the collection of data on behaviors that occur extremely infrequently,* such that they are likely to be missed in *in vivo* observations of behavior unless such observations are extended over exceptionally long periods of time.

• *Rating scales can gather information in ways that protect an individual's privacy,* apart from the topic of the rating scale itself. In contrast, direct observations or testing of the individual can prove exceptionally intrusive into the individual's daily life, giving the examiner the opportunity to witness situations and events that have no bearing on the topic or objective of the evaluation.

• *Rating scales are much less expensive, less time-consuming, and hence more efficient and cost-effective* than either tests or direct behavioral observation methods for many clinical and research purposes.

• *Rating scales may have normative data available for establishing the statistical deviance or relative position of the individual within the population concerning a behavior or trait of interest that may not be available for other methods of assessing that behavior or trait.* In the case of EF, such normative data can be less costly to collect than is the case for many tests of EF whose norms, if available at all, are typically not representative of large samples of the general population.

• *Rating scales can incorporate a large number of items that represent a given dimension, behavior, or trait, if so desired, that can be captured in a far less time-consuming format than can equivalent items within a psychological test.*

• *Rating scales can easily be used to collect the judgments of another who knows the index person well for comparison to the person's self-ratings as a means of judging interobserver agreement or the validity of the self-ratings.* Such judgments are far more difficult and cumbersome (if possible at all) for the results of a test, short of having a second examiner readminister the same test battery to the same person under the same or similar circumstances.

• *Rating scales can be used to filter out situational variation that has little or no bearing on the purpose of the evaluation* by asking for cross-situational judgments of the frequency, intensity, timing, or other aspects of the topography of the behavior under study. Again, these would be difficult if not impossible to achieve via a test or direct observational method.

• *Rating scales permit quantitative distinctions to be made concerning the qualitative aspects of human behavior* that are often difficult to obtain through other means, such as tests and observations, at least in a cost-effective manner.

• *Rating scales, like tests and observations, can be used for many different purposes.* These include subgrouping various populations along a trait or behavior of interest in epidemiological research; further exploring etiological hypotheses concerning certain behaviors or disorders; determining the prognosis of clinical groups of patients followed over long time intervals; and serving as measures of behavior change that may be secondary either to interventions or to a change in an individual's status, such as evaluating the consequences of various forms of brain injury or the impact of psychiatric disorders or psychological adversities.

For these and other reasons, behavior ratings of EF and its deficits in daily life activities have an important role to play in research and clinical practice in various psychological specialties.

Early Developmental History of the BDEFS

The development of the BDEFS has spanned more than a decade. The scale began originally as an attempt to evaluate EF in adults with ADHD, given the substantial research indicating that the disorder was associated with EF deficits on EF tests, at least at the group level of analysis (Frazier et al., 2004; Hervey et al., 2004). To assess EF deficits in daily life, my colleagues and I developed our own scale.

One other EF rating scale for adults existed at the time: the Dysexecutive Questionnaire (DEX; Burgess et al., 1998; Chaytor et al., 2006; Wood & Liossi, 2006). Though a commendable effort at creating a rating scale for EF deficits, it had several notable limitations that led us to develop our own EF scale (Barkley & Murphy, 2010b). The DEX comprised just 20 items meant to sample the broad range of symptoms believed to be representative of a general dysexecutive (frontal lobe) syndrome. This limited item pool was also not theoretically based but clinically based in its construction, originating in clinical descriptions of patients with PFC injuries. The scale did not yield scores concerning specific EF problem dimensions, but merely provided a single global summary score believed to reflect the dysexecutive syndrome.

A prototype EF scale (Barkley & Murphy, 2010b) was therefore developed for use in two large federally funded research projects on adults with ADHD (Barkley, Murphy, & Fischer, 2008). One of these projects, known as the UMASS Study, examined clinic-referred adults diagnosed with ADHD in comparison to both Clinical and Community control groups. The second study, known as the Milwaukee Study, was a follow-up study of hyperactive children into young adulthood (mean age 27). (See Barkley et al., 2008, for details of both studies.)

The scale's development was largely based on an earlier theory of EF, its five constructs, and their specific adaptive purposes (Barkley, 1997a, 1997b, 2001; see Chapter 1), as well as the larger literature on the nature of EF (see Denckla, 1996; Fuster, 1997; Lyon & Krasnegor, 1996; Stuss & Benson, 1986) and the rich and lengthy history of descriptions of the symptoms of patients with PFC injuries (again, see Chapter 1). The original item pool consisted of 91 items, which were developed to reflect inhibition; nonverbal working memory (self-directed sensing, especially visual imagery, sense of time, and time management); verbal working memory (self-directed private speech, verbal contemplation of one's behavior before acting, etc.); emotional/motivational self-regulation (inhibiting emotion, motivating oneself during boring activities, etc.); and reconstitution (generativity, planning, problem solving, and goal-directed inventiveness). According to this theory, the constructs are interactive and serve the overarching purpose of self-organizing behavior across time to prepare for and attain future goals. Items were also generated from a review of more than 200 charts of adults diagnosed with ADHD at a regional medical center's adult ADHD clinic, given that ADHD is largely a disorder of PFC functioning

(Bush, Valera, & Seidman, 2005; Hutchinson, Mathias, & Banich, 2008; Mackie et al., 2007; Paloyelis, Mehta, Kuntsi, & Asherson, 2007; Valera, Faraone, Murray, & Seidman, 2007), has long been construed as such (Pontius, 1973), and is characterized by many theorists as a disorder involving EF (Barkley, 1997b; Castellanos et al., 2006; Nigg & Casey, 2005; Sagvolden, Johansen, Aase, & Russell, 2005).

The scale items focused on problematic symptoms (deficit measurement) rather than on positive or normative EF functioning. The BDEFS was and is not intended to assess the broad variation of EF in the general population, in order to identify the range of individual differences in normal functioning that may exist in that population. Scales focusing on typical EF in a general population may be quite useful in studying the range of individual differences, as in studies of behavior genetics, normal development across the lifespan, or other purposes in which normal variation in a psychological trait is of interest. The BDEFS, in contrast, was and is intended to be used for clinical purposes, to evaluate the range of EF deficits in clinic-referred or high-risk adults—in other words, to assess symptoms of executive dysfunctioning. The clinician is faced with the question of the extent to which the complaints of a clinical patient concerning problems in EF are indicative of significant difficulties in EF. The question here is how atypical the patient's complaints are, rather than where the person falls within the distribution of normal variation in EF in the general population.

Deficit or symptom measurement is typical in the development of clinical assessment devices such as those used to assess anxiety, depression, bipolar disorders, or other adult psychological disorders—for instance, instruments such as the Symptom Checklist 90—Revised (SCL-90-R; Derogatis, 1986), or other rating scales of EF (e.g., Roth, Isquith, & Gioia, 2005). The distribution of such scores on symptom checklists will be quite different from the more typical bell-shaped curve of the distribution of normal variation in a typical psychological ability, such as intelligence or academic achievement. The score distribution of a deficit (symptom) measurement tool can be expected to have a distribution highly skewed toward the zero point or low score on the scale, with a steep drop in the percentage of the general population that manifests an increasing number of symptoms. Deficit or symptom assessment evaluates the likelihood that a patient's complaints are sufficiently severe or numerous to place the patient significantly outside the distribution of typical complaints for the general population. This was our purpose in constructing the BDEFS: to use items reflecting symptoms or deficits, rather than items reflecting the range of normal abilities.

Three separate instruments were developed from the original 91-item pool: two rating scales, and an interview to be given by a clinician. First, the 91 items were cast in the form of a rating scale to be completed by each participant. This scale was then recast in a third-person form to be completed by someone who knew the participant well. This was typically a parent or cohabiting partner, but if neither of these was available, a sibling or a close friend was used instead. Each item on these two scales was answered on a 0–3 Likert scale (0 = rarely or not at all, 1 = sometimes, 2 = often, and 3 = very often). The remainder of this chapter focuses mainly on these two rating scales, which served as the prototypes for the scales published in the present volume. Nevertheless, the participants in the UMASS Study also completed the interview with a clinical psychologist. The interview contained the same items as did the rating scale. The measures differed, however, in that the interview items asked only whether an individual had experienced that symptom as occurring often or more frequently during the past 6 months (see Barkley et al., 2008), rather than being given a choice of four possible ratings, as was the case with the rating scale. The term "often" was chosen to signify a symptom because of our earlier work with an adult ADHD rating scale, which suggested that this response occurs infrequently in the general population of adults to serve as a marker for a problem or symptom (Barkley & Murphy, 2006; Murphy & Barkley, 1996).

Three groups of participants (ages 18–60 years) were used in the initial UMASS Study of adults with ADHD (see Barkley et al., 2008; Barkley & Murphy, 2010b): (1) 146 adults clinically diagnosed with ADHD; (2) a Clinical control group (97 adults evaluated at the same clinic but not diagnosed with ADHD); and (3) a Community control group (109 adult volunteers from the local community). The adults in the first two groups were obtained from consecutive referrals to an adult ADHD clinic in a department of psychiatry at a regional medical school. The Community adults were obtained from advertisements posted throughout the medical school and from periodic newspaper ads in the regional newspaper. (More information on all three of these samples can be found in Barkley et al., 2008.) Slightly more than two-thirds (68%) of those in our group with ADHD were males; this differed from a nearly equal sex distribution (51%) in our Community control group, but was not significantly different from the distribution in the Clinical control group (56%). This finding is in keeping with many studies of children and adults with ADHD, which demonstrate a greater representation of the disorder in males than in females (Barkley, 2006; Kessler et al., 2006). Typically, the male–female ratio in ADHD is approximately 2:1 in adult epidemiological studies—a ratio similar to that found here. The vast majority of participants were White (94%), or of European American ancestry, and the groups did not differ in this respect. Therefore, caution is warranted in extrapolating the initial results described below to adults in other ethnic groups.

We had ratings from others on 129 (88%) of the group with ADHD, 88 (90%) of the Clinical group, and 92 (84%) of the Community group. These differences in the percentage of each group having collateral reports of EF were not significant ($\chi^2 = 19.38$, $df = 12$, $p =$ NS). Examination of the pattern of relationships of these other people to the participants revealed no significant differences across the groups.

Identifying Underlying Dimensions of EF in Daily Life Activities

We applied principal-components factor analysis to the 91 original items in the prototype of the BDEFS (hereafter referred to as the P-BDEFS) to explore the underlying dimensions of EF deficits in daily life, using self-reports from the entire UMASS sample of 352 participants. This gave us 3.86 participants per EF item on the scale, which was below the traditionally recommended 5 participants per variable to achieve adequate reliability of the factor structure. Nevertheless, as noted below, evidence for the actual reliability of this factor structure was obtained from the fact that the same factor structure emerged from the other-report ratings of EF deficits in this study. It also emerged in the Milwaukee Study, the separate study of hyperactive children followed to adulthood, which used the interview version of this rating scale (Barkley & Fischer, in press). Finally, it emerged in the subsequent version of the BDEFS with the normative sample to be discussed in Chapter 3 (N = 1,249).

Although 10 factors were obtained that had eigenvalues greater than 1, only five of these had at least 10 items with their highest loading on a factor; accounted for at least 2% or more of the variance before rotation; and, incidentally, had eigenvalues of 1.8 or higher. We therefore retained just those five factors. We found that 88 items had loadings of at least .400 on any of these five factors. Three items were dropped from the scale because they did not have a loading of ≥ .400 on any of the final five factors in that analysis ("Can't seem to sustain friendships or close relationships as long as other people," "Poor or sloppy handwriting," and "Less able than others to recall events from childhood").

The unrotated factor solution indicated that the first factor accounted for a substantial amount of the variance in these ratings (over 51%). Each of the remaining factors accounted for 2–4.4% of the variance per factor, such that the five unrotated factors explained more than 63% of the variance. It appeared that one large factor accounted for the majority of variance in EF deficits in daily life. A similar finding was evident in the factor analyses of the Behavior Rating Inventory of Executive Functioning (BRIEF)—Adult Version (Roth et al., 2005). An identical finding was noted by Biederman and colleagues (2008), using the P-BDEFS with a different sample of adults who had ADHD and control adults. The highest-loading items on this first factor for the P-BDEFS dealt with sense of time, time management, planning, preparing for deadlines, and other goal-directed behavior. We therefore labeled this factor as Self-Management to Time. Such a finding supports the view of Fuster (1997) and others (see Chapter 1) that EF chiefly comprises the cross-temporal organization of behavior toward goals.

Many investigators might have stopped the analysis with these findings, concluding that EF in daily life activities chiefly comprises this single dimension. An identical finding was noted by Faraone and colleagues (2010). However, another 12% of the variance (prior to rotation) could be accounted for by four additional factors that each accounted for at least 2% or more of the unrotated variance; had at least 10 items loading primarily on that dimension; and, incidentally, had eigenvalues of at least 1.8. The issue concerning the number of items assigned to a factor is important if a dimension is to have any chance of being assessed reliably; reliability (as well as validity) is in part dependent on the number of items for a construct included in the scale. And so we subsequently used a varimax rotation to analyze the scale further, specifying a five-factor solution. (A promax rotation yielded the same results, except that the factor loadings of the items were even higher than those found in the varimax rotation. This was to be expected, given the purposes of each approach to rotation. Varimax seeks to decrease correlations among the factors, whereas promax permits such correlations to exist across factors.) The final five factors for the self-report version of the P-BDEFS, and their variance (after the varimax rotation), were as follows:

- *Factor 1* (*Self-Management to Time*) contained 23 items and accounted for 15.7% of the variance after rotation. As noted above, the highest-loading items dealt with sense of time, time management, planning, preparing for deadlines, and other goal-directed behavior.
- *Factor 2* (*Self-Organization/Problem Solving*) contained 21 items and accounted for 15.2% of the variance. The highest-loading items pertained to organizing one's thoughts, actions, and writing; thinking quickly when encountering unexpected events; and inventing solutions to problems or obstacles encountered while pursuing goals.
- *Factor 3* (*Self-Restraint or Inhibition*) comprised 23 items and accounted for 14.1% of the variance. Its highest-loading items dealt with making impulsive comments, poor inhibition of reactions to events, impulsive decision making, doing things without regard to their consequences, and not thinking about the relevant past or future before acting. A few items also dealt with poor self-awareness and the inability to take other people's perspectives about their own behavior or a situation.
- *Factor 4* (*Self-Motivation*) consisted of 11 items and accounted for 9.8% of the variance, with items mainly dealing with taking short cuts in one's work, not doing all assigned work, being described as lazy by others, not putting in much effort on work, needing more supervision than others while working, getting bored easily, and so forth.
- *Factor 5* (*Self-Activation/Concentration*) contained 10 items and explained 8.6% of the variance. It comprised items dealing with being easily distracted by one's thoughts when doing boring work; staying awake and alert while working; being able to persist at boring activities; sustained concentration in reading, paperwork, meetings, or other activities that were not interesting; being prone to daydreaming when one should be concentrating; and having to reread uninteresting written material in order to comprehend it.

As noted above, a factor analysis with varimax rotation was also conducted on the version of the P-BDEFS completed by others (Barkley & Murphy, 2010b). The same five-factor solution emerged with nearly identical item content. The variance accounted for after rotation by each factor was as follows: Self-Management to Time, 19.9%; Self-Organization/Problem Solving, 16.5%; Self-Restraint, 16.7%; Self-Motivation, 8%; and Self-Activation/Concentration, 3.8%. In only a few instances did an item have its highest loading on a factor different from the one to which it was assigned in the self-ratings. Even then, it had either an equivalent loading or a second-highest loading on the scale to which it was assigned in the self-ratings. It is important to note here that the P-BDEFS was limited by the absence of any items addressing the domain of emotional self-regulation. Therefore, there was no opportunity for such a factor to emerge in these analyses. This limitation was corrected in the final version of the BDEFS, as described in the next section.

We created five subscales from the self-report version of the P-BDEFS reflecting these factors and consisting of just those items having their highest loading on each subscale. For each subscale, we created a total score based on the sum of the individual raw item scores. We did the same for the other-report version, using the identical items, so that direct comparisons could be made between the two versions.

Despite the emergence of these five factor-based subscales on the P-BDEFS, the subscales were significantly intercorrelated, ranging from .74 to .88 for the self-ratings and .75 to .88 for the other-ratings. The subscales therefore shared 56–77% of their variance, which, as suggested above and in Chapter 1, may indicate the possible existence of a single underlying metaconstruct of deficits in EF (Barkley & Murphy, 2010b).

For the self-ratings, three of the five subscales showed a low but significant correlation with participant age: Self-Management to Time ($r = -.11$, $p = .05$); Self-Motivation ($r = -.21$, $p < .001$); and Self-Activation ($r = -.11$, $p = .04$). This was true for these same three subscales rated by others: Self-Management to Time ($r = -.16$, $p = .01$); Self-Motivation ($r = -.27$, $p < .001$); and Self-Activation ($r = -.16$, $p = .009$) (Barkley & Murphy, 2010b). Thus older individuals within the age range of this study had fewer deficits in EF in daily life.

Only one of the five self-rating subscales was modestly but significantly correlated with participant IQ: Self-Organization/Problem Solving ($r = -.15$, $p = .007$). This pattern was also the case for the other-ratings ($r = -.17$, $p = .008$) (Barkley & Murphy, 2010b). These results suggest that, unlike EF tests, ratings of EF in daily life activities are largely not contaminated by general intelligence. Even the single subscale that was related to intelligence shared just 2.9% of its variance with the IQ measure used in our study.

Our results indicated that the adults with ADHD rated themselves as having significantly more severe EF deficits on all five subscales, compared to both the Clinical and Community control groups. The adults in the Clinical group also rated themselves as having more severe EF deficits than the Community group. This was also the case for the other-ratings.

We also used the Community control group to determine a threshold for being clinically deficient on each of the five subscales. We specified this deficiency as being +1.5 standard deviations above the mean of that group on the P-BDEFS. For self-reports, we found that 89–98% of the group with ADHD and 83–93% of the Clinical group fell into this clinically significant range (7th percentile of the Community group), compared to just 7–11% of the Community group, on the five subscales of the P-BDEFS. The ADHD group had a significantly greater percentage thus impaired on the Self-Motivation scale than the Clinical group, but these differences were not significant on the other subscales. When other-ratings were used, the figures were 84–99% of the ADHD group and 68–89% of the Clinical group, compared to 9–14% of the Community group. The ADHD group had a higher percentage rated as impaired by others on four of the five subscales, the exception being Self-Organization/Problem Solving.

Adult ADHD was therefore associated with significant deficits in EF in daily life as assessed by the P-BDEFS, and the majority of those adults were in the clinically deficient range in EF in daily life (Barkley & Murphy, 2010b). These results indicated that the P-BDEFS could readily distinguish clinic-referred patients having a psychiatric diagnosis from nonclinical controls; in fact, the two distributions of scores (clinic vs. nonclinic) showed only limited overlap. Our research also found that adults with ADHD had the most severe deficits in the five dimensions of EF assessed by the scale relative to the Clinical controls, and that both of these groups manifested substantially more EF deficits than did the Community control group.

Using these factors and their item loadings, we computed the same scores for using the interview form of the P-BDEFS mentioned earlier. Again, these items were answered as yes (the item occurred often or more frequently) or no (the item did not occur often). The interview form therefore yielded the equivalent of an EF symptom count. For the present manual, the factor scores from the interview were correlated with those noted above for the P-BDEFS self-report rating scale. The results showed that the scores for each of the factors were highly correlated between these two measures: Self-Management to Time ($r = .921$), Self-Organization/Problem Solving (.885), Self-Restraint (.873), Self-Motivation (.867), Self-Activation/Concentration (.904), and the Total EF Summary Score (sum of all factor scores) (.925). All correlations were significant at $p < .001$. Given the high magnitude of these relationships, it is likely that any of the findings discussed here and in Chapters 6 and 7 (on reliability and validity of the BDEFS rating scale) would apply just as much to the interview form.

This became evident when the interview was used in a subsequent study with different samples: In the Milwaukee Study, the separate study of hyperactive children followed to adulthood, we found the same factor structure for the interview version of the P-BDEFS (Barkley & Fischer, in press). Children whose ADHD had persisted to age 27 years were found to have significantly more EF deficits in daily life than were such children whose ADHD had not persisted. And the latter group had more severe EF deficits than did the Community control group followed to adulthood. Thus, again, we found that persistence of ADHD into adulthood was associated with more severe EF deficits in daily life activities, and that by adulthood more severe ADHD was linked to more severe EF deficits. Such findings have also been reported in research on children with ADHD by investigators using several different rating scales of EF (Gioia, Isquith, Kenworthy, & Barton, 2002; Thorell, Eninger, Brocki, & Bohlin, 2010).

The P-BDEFS thus appeared to have utility for the clinical assessment of EF in daily life activities. The initial scale assessed five dimensions of EF deficits in daily life activities and was found to be useful in identifying such deficits in adults diagnosed with ADHD and other clinically referred adults relative to a Community group, as well as in children with ADHD followed to adulthood. This led us to proceed with further development of the scale, the collection of norms for the present BDEFS, and publication of that information in this manual.

Further Development of the BDEFS

For the BDEFS rating scales published in this manual, the items from the P-BDEFS that were found to have factor loadings of at least .500 or greater on one of the five factors in our earlier study (Barkley & Murphy, 2010b) were retained. Therefore, a few items on each of the P-BDEFS subscales were abandoned, in an attempt to reduce the overall scale's length and hence the time needed to complete it without loss of information on the five subscales. A further examination of the scale items, as well as the resulting factor structure, suggested that one domain of EF appeared to be substantially underrepresented in the P-BDEFS and so did not have an opportunity to emerge in the foregoing analyses. This component was the self-regulation of emotion. The few items on the prototype scale that dealt with emotion were primarily representing the impulsive expression of impatience, frustration, and anger, and loaded on the Self-Restraint (Inhibition) factor, as might be expected. But there were no items pertaining to self-management of emotion on the P-BDEFS. This is an important component of EF that is often neglected in developing EF test batteries, but appears to be commonly observed among the deficits in clinical patients with PFC injuries (see Chapter 1).

Emotional self-control is believed to comprise a two-stage process: (1) the inhibition of strong emotional reactions to events; and (2) the subsequent engagement of self-regulatory actions and strategies that include (a) self-soothing, (b) refocusing attention away from the provocative event, (c) reducing and moderating the initial emotion, and (d) organizing the eventual emotional expression so that it is more consistent with and supportive of individual goals and long-term welfare (Barkley, 2010; Gottman & Katz, 1989; Hinshaw, 2003; Martel, 2009; Masters, 1991; Melnick & Hinshaw, 2000). It is argued that deficits in both of these components of emotional self-control lead to impulsive emotional expression and the subsequent deficient self-regulation of those emotions in conformity with personal or social purposes and goals.

I used the model of emotional self-regulation developed by Gross (1998; Gross & John, 2003; Gross & Thompson, 2007) to generate an additional 10 items to reflect these problems with poor self-regulation of emotional states, as well as two additional items related to self-motivation. This was done in an effort to strengthen (lengthen) the item content of the Self-Motivation subscale in the P-BDEFS. Gross and Thompson (2007) have argued that there are five sets of emotion regulation strategies: situation selection, situation modification, attention deployment (such as distraction or gaze aversion), cognitive change (such as conscious reappraisal), and response modulation (such as suppressing expressions). These five sets of strategies can be further subdivided by whether they are antecedent-focused or response-focused. Efforts were made to have at least one item in the BDEFS evaluate each of these strategies.

The final version of the BDEFS on which the national norms would be collected therefore contained 100 items. Following further analyses to be reported later in this manual, the final scale was reduced to 89 items. And from that scale, a shorter version was also developed, comprising 20 items having the highest loadings on their respective factors. With this background information, the survey methods used to collect normative data on the scale and the demographic characteristics of that sample are presented in the next chapter.

CHAPTER 3

Normative Sample

The Self-Report version of the full BDEFS was normed on a large, nationally representative sample of adults in the United States ages 18–70+, with equal representation of males and females in each of four regions. To do this, a national survey company, Knowledge Networks of Menlo Park, California, was hired (see its website, *knowledgenetworks.com*, for more information on the company).

Methods

Knowledge Networks conducted the survey by using the Web-enabled Knowledge Panel®, a probability-based panel designed to be representative of the U.S. population. Initially, participants were chosen scientifically by a random selection of telephone numbers and residential addresses. Persons in selected households were then invited by telephone or by mail to participate in the Knowledge Panel®. For those who agreed to participate but did not already have Internet access, Knowledge Networks provided at no cost a laptop and Internet service provider connection. People who already had computers and Internet service were permitted to use their own equipment to participate. Panelists then received unique log-in information for accessing surveys online, and then were sent emails throughout each month inviting them to participate in research. Panelists were paid for their completion of the survey. More technical information is available on the website mentioned above (*knowledgenetworks.com/ganp/reviewer-info.html*).

The initial 100-item BDEFS was given to Knowledge Networks as a rating scale in which respondents were to answer each item on a 4-point (1–4) Likert scale: 1 = rarely or not at all, 2 = sometimes, 3 = often, and 4 = very often. The scale was then uploaded to an Internet site, and members of the Knowledge Panel® were invited to complete the scale. The interview version was not used in this study. The survey was conducted in April 2010 and was completed within 3 weeks of the initial invitation. The company was contracted to obtain completed scales on at least 1,200 adults divided into six age groups (18–29, 30–39, 40–49, 50–59, 60–69, and 70+), with at least 100 males and 100 females in each age group. A subset of participants were invited to complete the survey a second time, 2–3 weeks after the initial scale was completed, to provide information for computing test–retest reliability. A total of 62 participants, 31 males and 31 females, did so. They were randomly selected to ensure that at least five males and five females were drawn from each age group. Like the initial participants, these returning participants were paid for their time in completing this second administration.

Norms were not collected for the Other-Report version of the full BDEFS, as there was no means available in this process by which such a sample of others could be obtained conveniently. This would have required every participant to have someone available and willing to complete that version of the scale. In addition, these others would have had (1) to be provided with Internet access if necessary, (2) to be available in equal numbers that fell within the same types of relationships to the participants, (3) to have similar levels of experience with the participants, and (4) to be representative of the U.S. Census. In particular, past research shows that the nature of the relationship between a participant and a collateral person providing information about him or her has significant effects on the degree of agreement and amount of disparities in the ratings (Barkley et al., in press). For these and other reasons, no effort was made to collect norms for the Other-Report version. Finally, the important issue in obtaining reports from others is not how their reports compare to those of a normative group of collateral informants providing such reports, but how their reports differ from those of the patients/participants. The reports of others about index persons do not constitute a check on the statistical deviance of individuals within the population, but a check on the validity of the participants' own reports about themselves.

Knowledge Networks requires that participants be given the option of choosing not to answer a question. For most questions, this did not occur. However, for some questions, a rare participant did refuse to answer the question. For each of the questions for which refusals occurred, this occurred between 1 and 12 times, with an average of 4 such refused replies for such questions. This constitutes a refusal rate of 0.1–0.9% for those items on which this occurred, with an average rate of less than 0.3%. In these rare cases, the missing answer was replaced with a 1 (the lowest rating), so that all of the remaining data for this participant could be used in the project. This practice was based on the argument that this would create a conservative bias in the responses to that item.

Several differences between this approach to collecting norms for an EF rating scale and that used for the adult form of the BRIEF are worth noting here. The manual for the adult BRIEF (Roth et al., 2005) indicates that a representative sample of the all U.S. adults was not obtained; instead, only those who had Internet access were invited. This approach can bias the resulting sample away from the general U.S. population, a substantial subset of which do not routinely have access to the Internet and/or do not own computer equipment. The approach used here sampled U.S. adults regardless of their Internet access and provided such access to those adults who did not otherwise have such access or the necessary computer equipment. Another important distinction is that the BRIEF developers excluded anyone (1) with a psychiatric diagnosis, (2) with self-reported use of a psychiatric drug, (3) with a learning disability, (4) with a neurological disorder, or (5) with a serious medical illness. A substantial minority of the U.S. population (usually cited as 20–25%) qualifies for a psychiatric disorder alone, and probably many more qualify for these other rule-out developmental and medical disorders. A sample thus filtered is not representative of the general U.S. population, but of a psychiatrically and medically nondisordered population. Comparison of any patient's results to such a sample would make it far more likely that the individual's scores might deviate from this ultranormal normative sample than from one based on the general U.S. population regardless of presence of various disorders or history of treatment, as was done here. The issue of a person's relative position within the general population would seem to require comparison to a representative sample of that entire adult population, rather than to a sample including only psychiatrically and medically healthy individuals who are not so representative.

Demographic Characteristics of the National Sample

A total of 1,249 adults completed the survey. The sample sizes for each age group by sex are shown in Table 3.1, along with the percentage of the entire sample each represented. They indicate that the survey methods were successful in obtaining an equal representation of males and females at each of the six age groups requested of Knowledge Networks.

TABLE 3.1. The Numbers of Males and Females in Six Age Groups in the BDEFS Normative Sample

Sex and age group	Frequency	Percent	Cumulative percent
Male 18–29	104	8.3	8.3
Male 30–39	102	8.2	16.5
Male 40–49	104	8.3	24.8
Male 50–59	104	8.3	33.1
Male 60–69	104	8.3	41.5
Male 70+	105	8.4	49.9
Female 18–29	102	8.2	58.0
Female 30–39	104	8.3	66.4
Female 40–49	105	8.4	74.8
Female 50–59	106	8.5	83.3
Female 60–69	105	8.4	91.7
Female 70+	104	8.3	100.0
Total	1,249	100.0	

A total of 623 males ages 18–93 years (49.9%) and 626 females ages 18–96 years completed the sample. However, just 10 participants were older than 87 years. The mean age for males was 49.7 years (SD = 18.0), and for females was 49.8 years (SD = 18.0); these were not significantly different (F = 0.003, p = NS). (Note that henceforth, statistical significance for the demographic factors is set at $p \leq .05$.) The 2000 U.S. Census indicated that 49.1% of the U.S. population was male, and thus our sample's sex distribution approximated that of the United States generally. Nearly equal numbers of males and females were placed into four educational categories, so that the sexes did not differ in their educational levels (χ^2 = 0.60, p = NS), as shown in Table 3.2. The educational levels of the normative sample were also generally comparable to those of the U.S. population as reflected in the 2000 U.S. Census, although the normative sample contained a slightly lower percentage of those with less than a high school education than was the case for the U.S. Census.

The geographic distribution of the participants within each sex is shown in Table 3.3. As this table indicates, males and females in the study were obtained from all four regions of the United States in relatively equal proportions. There was no significant difference in the geographic distributions as a function of participants' sex (χ^2 = 3.12, p = NS). The results show that the geographic distribution of the normative sample was quite similar to that of the U.S. population, based on the 2000 U.S. Census.

The racial/ethnic breakdown of the normative sample by sex is displayed in Table 3.4. As seen in that table, the majority of the participants were White (non-Hispanic), as was the case in 2000 in the U.S. population. There were no significant differences in the ethnic breakdown of the sample for each sex (χ^2 = 2.34, p = NS). The percentage of participants in each ethnic group resembled to a large extent that for the U.S. population, based on the 2000 U.S. Census. However, blacks and Hispanics appeared to be slightly underrepresented in the normative sample.

TABLE 3.2. Education Levels for Each Sex in the Normative Sample, in Comparison to the 2000 U.S. Census

Education category		Sex			Percent of
		Male	Female	Total	U.S. Census[a]
Less than high school	Count	73	69	142	
	% within gender	11.7%	11.0%	11.4%	19.6%
High school	Count	178	190	368	
	% within gender	28.6%	30.4%	29.5%	28.6%
Some college	Count	182	183	365	
	% within gender	29.2%	29.2%	29.2%	21.0%
Bachelor's degree or higher	Count	190	184	374	
	% within gender	30.5%	29.4%	29.9%	24.1%

[a]Based on the 2000 U.S. Census (available at *www.census.gov*).

TABLE 3.3. Regional Distribution by Sex for the Normative Sample, in Comparison to the 2000 U.S. Census

Region		Sex: Male	Sex: Female	Total	Percent of U.S. Census[a]
Northeast	Count	111	126	237	
	% within gender	17.8%	20.1%	19.0%	19.0%
Midwest	Count	133	150	283	
	% within gender	21.3%	24.0%	22.7%	22.9%
South	Count	237	219	456	
	% within gender	38.0%	35.0%	36.5%	35.6%
West	Count	142	131	273	
	% within gender	22.8%	20.9%	21.9%	22.4%

[a]Based on the 2000 U.S. Census (available at *www.census.gov*).

TABLE 3.4. Frequency and Percentage of Each Racial/Ethnic Group by Sex for the Normative Sample, in Comparison to the 2000 U.S. Census

Race/ethnic group		Sex: Male	Sex: Female	Total	Percent of U.S. Census[a]
White non-Hispanic	Count	478	488	966	
	% within gender	76.7%	78.0%	77.3%	75.1%
Black non-Hispanic	Count	43	42	85	
	% within gender	6.9%	6.7%	6.8%	12.3%
Other non-Hispanic	Count	20	27	47	
	% within gender	3.2%	4.3%	3.8%	6.6%
Hispanic	Count	61	50	111	
	% within gender	9.8%	8.0%	8.9%	12.5%
2+ races, non-Hispanic	Count	21	19	40	
	% within gender	3.4%	3.0%	3.2%	2.4%
Total		623	626	1,249	

[a]Based on the 2000 U.S. Census (available at *www.census.gov*).

The breakdown of the normative sample by income categories is shown in Table 3.5. The mean income category was 11.3, which translated into a mean income ranging from $40,000 to $49,999; the median category was 12, equivalent to an income ranging from $50,000 to $59,999. The modal income category was 13, reflecting a range of $60,000–69,999. The median U.S. household income was $41,994 as of the 2000 U.S. Census. The results suggest a relatively reasonable resemblance of the normative sample's household income to that of the U.S. population.

The marital status of the normative sample participants is shown in Table 3.6. It suggests a reasonable similarity between the normative sample and the U.S. population, based on the 2000 U.S. Census. However, a somewhat lower percentage of the normative sample appeared to have never been married than was the case in the U.S. Census. The U.S. Census Bureau computes marital status for persons 15 years of age and older, which would of course reflect a higher percentage having never been married than was the case for the normative sample, which included individuals 18 years of age and older. We would expect more of the latter group to be married, relative to the U.S. Census method of determining this figure. This probably explains the difference in marital status between the U.S. Census data and those for the normative sample.

The employment status of the normative sample is shown in Table 3.7. More than half of those in the sample were working as paid employees or in self-employment, and nearly a quarter of the respondents were in retirement. The 2000 U.S. Census

TABLE 3.5. Distribution of Household Income Categories for the Normative Sample

Income category	Frequency	Percent	Cumulative percent
Less than $5,000	18	1.4	1.4
$5,000 to $7,499	21	1.7	3.1
$7,500 to $9,999	27	2.2	5.3
$10,000 to $12,499	36	2.9	8.2
$12,500 to $14,999	35	2.8	11.0
$15,000 to $19,999	55	4.4	15.4
$20,000 to $24,999	63	5.0	20.4
$25,000 to $29,999	70	5.6	26.0
$30,000 to $34,999	65	5.2	31.2
$35,000 to $39,999	79	6.3	37.6
$40,000 to $49,999	110	8.8	46.4
$50,000 to $59,999	116	9.3	55.6
$60,000 to $74,999	141	11.3	66.9
$75,000 to $84,999	89	7.1	74.1
$85,000 to $99,999	98	7.8	81.9
$100,000 to $124,999	99	7.9	89.8
$125,000 to $149,999	52	4.2	94.0
$150,000 to $174,999	36	2.9	96.9
$175,000 or more	39	3.1	100.0

TABLE 3.6. Marital Status of the Normative Sample, in Comparison to the 2000 U.S. Census

Marital status	Frequency	Percent	Percent of U.S. Census[a]
Married	659	52.8	54.4
Widowed	85	6.8	6.6
Divorced	118	9.4	9.7
Separated	28	2.2	2.2
Never married	264	21.1	27.1
Living with partner	95	7.6	—

[a]Based on the 2000 U.S. Census (available at *www.census.gov*).

figure for those currently employed was 57.5% for individuals 16 years of age and older. This indicates a reasonable similarity of the normative sample to the U.S. population in terms of employment status.

To summarize the demographic characteristics of the study sample, it appears that the normative sample recruited here closely approximated the U.S. adult population as reflected in the 2000 U.S. Census concerning regional distribution, sex, race/ethnic group, marital status, employment status, total household income, and education. This was the normative sample on which data from the initial 100-item version of the BDEFS were collected. The results for the factor analyses of the scale and construction of the individual subscales based on this normative sample's responses are discussed in the next chapter.

TABLE 3.7. Employment Status of the Normative Sample

Employment status	Frequency	Percent	Cumulative percent
Working—as a paid employee	573	45.9	45.9
Working—self-employed	81	6.5	52.4
Not working—on temporary layoff from a job	20	1.6	54.0
Not working—looking for work	90	7.2	61.2
Not working—retired	282	22.6	83.7
Not working—disabled	99	7.9	91.7
Not working—other	104	8.3	100.0
Total	1,249	100.0	

CHAPTER 4

Factor Analysis, Scale Construction, and Item Frequencies

This chapter reports the results of the factor analysis intended to uncover the underlying dimensions of EF in daily life activities as assessed by the BDEFS. It then discusses the use of those results to construct the final version and subscales of the BDEFS. Finally, a table showing the frequencies with which the items were endorsed by the normative sample is presented and discussed.

Factor Analysis

The initial 100-item version of the BDEFS was submitted to a principal-components factor analysis (PCFA), using the entire normative sample of 1,249 adults described in Chapter 3. The initial results revealed that 13 factors had eigenvalues greater than 1. However, each of these factors accounted for only 1.0–1.6% of the variance and contained only a few items. They were therefore considered to be unreliable and of little clinical interest. Another six factors were found to have eigenvalues greater than 2 and to account for at least 2% of the variance each. However, the last factor (Factor 6) had only four items that had their highest loading on this factor and loaded at least .400 after varimax rotation. This factor was associated with some of the items from the original Self-Activation/Concentration factor discovered in the initial research on the P-BDEFS, discussed in Chapter 2. The remaining five factors each contained at least 12 items that had their highest loadings on that factor, had factor loadings of at least .400 or higher after varimax rotation (or .500 after promax rotation), and accounted for at least 2.5% of the variance each.

The results were then submitted initially to a varimax rotation, which is designed to maximize as many values in each column of the factor-loading coefficient table as close to zero as possible. This approach is typically used in an attempt to reduce the degree of correlation among the items (variables). But we also submitted the initial PCFA to a promax rotation, which is frequently used when variables are known to be correlated (as are the EF items) and allows items to be correlated with more than one factor. Both approaches yielded the same eventual factor structure. The results of the PCFA are shown in Table 4.1. It reports the factor loadings for both the varimax and promax rotations.

The first factor accounted for 37.0% of the variance before rotation and contained 15 of the items from the Self-Organization/Problem Solving factor found in the initial P-BDEFS (see Chapter 2), as well as six items from the initial Self-Activation/Concentration factor. As noted above, the latter factor was discarded in the present analysis because of a limited item set. This explains the likely reason for that finding, as it appears that many of the items that originally loaded on the Self-Activation/Concentration factor in the P-BDEFS moved to the Self-Organization/Problem Solving factor in the analysis of this much larger normative sample. Factor 1 therefore contained 24 items and was once again labeled as Self-Organization/Problem Solving. The seven highest-loading items, in descending order, were these:

- Have difficulty explaining things in their proper order or sequence
- I don't seem to process information as quickly or as accurately as others
- Have trouble learning new or complex activities as well as others
- Unable to "think on my feet" or respond as effectively as others to unexpected events
- Unable to come up with or invent as many solutions to problems as others seem to do
- I am slower than others at solving problems I encounter in my daily life
- Find myself at a loss for words when I want to explain something to others

Factor 2 accounted for 5.1% of the variance prior to rotation and contained 20 of the original 23 items from the Self-Management to Time factor discovered in the initial research with the P-BDEFS. It also contained an item that was originally found to load on the Self-Activation/Concentration factor, but no longer did so in this subsequent analysis using the larger normative sample. This factor thus had 21 items, and it was once again labeled as Self-Management to Time. The seven highest-loading items, again in descending order, were as follows:

- Can't seem to get things done unless there is an immediate deadline
- Not motivated to prepare in advance for things I know I am supposed to do
- Procrastinate or put off doing things until the last minute
- Waste or mismanage my time
- Have trouble doing what I tell myself to do
- Poor sense of time
- Have difficulty motivating myself to stick with my work and get it done

(text resumes on page 45)

TABLE 4.1. Rotated Factor Loadings for BDEFS Items Based on PCFA with Varimax (and Promax) Rotation

Factor name/scale items[a]	Factors 1	2	3	4	5
1. Self-Organization/Problem Solving					
EF23. I do not seem to anticipate the future as much or as well as others	.415 (.602)[b]				
EF24. Can't seem to remember what I previously heard or read about	.595 (.656)				
EF25. I have trouble organizing my thoughts	.590 (.739)				
EF26. When I am shown something complicated to do, I cannot keep the information in mind so as to imitate or do it correctly	.659 (.718)				
EF27. I have trouble considering various options for doing things and weighing their consequences	.631 (.747)				
EF28. Have difficulties saying what I want to say	.606 (.670)				
EF29. Unable to come up with or invent as many solutions to problems as others seem to do	.666 (.740)				
EF30. Find myself at a loss for words when I want to explain something to others	.665 (.714)				
EF31. Have trouble putting my thoughts down in writing as well or as quickly as others	.659 (.699)				
EF32. Feel I am not as creative or inventive as others of my level of intelligence	.558 (.629)				
EF33. In trying to accomplish goals or assignments, I find I am not able to think of as many ways of doing things as others	.646 (.729)				
EF34. Have trouble learning new or complex activities as well as others	.687 (.741)				
EF35. Have difficulty explaining things in their proper order or sequence	.741 (.785)				
EF36. Can't seem to get to the point of my explanations as quickly as others	.634 (.706)				
EF37. Have trouble doing things in their proper order or sequence	.659 (.756)				
EF38. Unable to "think on my feet" or respond as effectively as others to unexpected events	.672 (.736)				
EF39. I am slower than others at solving problems I encounter in my daily life	.666 (.777)				
EF76. Easily distracted by irrelevant events or thoughts when I must concentrate on something	.409 (.611)				
EF78. Not able to comprehend what I read as well as I should be able to do; have to reread material to get its meaning	.596 (.661)				
EF79. Cannot focus my attention on tasks or work as well as others	.520 (.705)				
EF82. Easily confused	.642 (.751)				
EF83. Can't seem to sustain my concentration on reading, paperwork, lectures, or work	.538 (.684)				

(cont.)

TABLE 4.1. *(cont.)*

Factor name/scale items[a]		Factors 1	2	3	4	5
EF89.	Find it hard to focus on what is important from what is not important when I do things	.484 (.705)				
EF90.	I don't seem to process information as quickly or as accurately as others	.689 (.780)				
2. Self-Management to Time						
EF1.	Procrastinate or put off doing things until the last minute		.676 (.691)			
EF2.	Poor sense of time		.653 (.691)			
EF3.	Waste or mismanage my time		.664 (.710)			
EF4.	Not prepared on time for work or assigned tasks		.632 (.700)			
EF5.	Fail to meet deadlines for assignments		.516 (.637)			
EF6.	Have trouble planning ahead or preparing for upcoming events		.622 (.715)			
EF7.	Forget to do things I am supposed to do		.562 (.650)			
EF8.	Can't seem to accomplish the goals I set for myself		.619 (.718)			
EF9.	Late for work or scheduled appointments		.577 (.622)			
EF10.	Can't seem to hold in mind things I need to remember to do		.523 (.653)			
EF11.	Can't seem to get things done unless there is an immediate deadline		.693 (.762)			
EF12.	Have difficulty judging how much time it will take to do something or get somewhere		.580 (.682)			
EF13.	Have trouble motivating myself to start work		.622 (.711)			
EF14.	Have difficulty motivating myself to stick with my work and get it done		.658 (.770)			
EF15.	Not motivated to prepare in advance for things I know I am supposed to do		.681 (.781)			
EF16.	Have trouble completing one activity before starting into a new one		.562 (.660)			
EF17.	Have trouble doing what I tell myself to do		.665 (.770)			
EF18.	Difficulties following through on promises or commitments I may make to others		.477 (.630)			
EF19.	Lack self-discipline		.582 (.703)			
EF20.	Have difficulty arranging or doing my work by its priority or importance; can't "prioritize" well		.597 (.749)			
EF80.	Find it hard to get started or get going on things I need to get done		.455 (.647)			

(cont.)

TABLE 4.1. *(cont.)*

Factor name/scale items[a]	Factors 1	2	3	4	5
3. Self-Restraint (Inhibition)					
EF40. Find it difficult to tolerate waiting; impatient			.452 (.592)		
EF41. Make decisions impulsively			.580 (.659)		
EF42. Unable to inhibit my reactions or responses to events or others			.584 (.690)		
EF43. Have difficulty stopping my activities or behavior when I should do so			.544 (.696)		
EF44. Have difficulty changing my behavior when I am given feedback about my mistakes			.522 (.663)		
EF45. Make impulsive comments to others			.625 (.693)		
EF46. Likely to do things without considering the consequences for doing them			.624 (.740)		
EF47. Change my plans at the last minute on a whim or last minute impulse			.482 (.563)		
EF48. Fail to consider past relevant events or past personal experiences before responding to situations (I act without thinking)			.587 (.735)		
EF49. Not aware of things I say or do			.473 (.641)		
EF50. Have difficulty being objective about things that affect me			.455 (.609)		
EF51. Find it hard to take other people's perspectives about a problem or situation			.523 (.637)		
EF54. Don't think about or talk things over with myself before doing something			.579 (.719)		
EF55. Trouble following the rules in a situation			.539 (.677)		
EF56. More likely to drive a motor vehicle much faster than others (Excessive speeding)			.481 (.513)		
EF57. Have a low tolerance for frustrating situations			.500 (.618)		
EF58. Cannot inhibit my emotions as well as others			.500 (.672)		
EF60. I don't look ahead and think about what the future outcomes will be before I do something (I don't use my foresight)			.522 (.698)		
EF61. I engage in risk taking activities more than others are likely to do			.505 (.580)		
4. Self-Regulation of Emotion					
EF52. Quick to get angry or become upset				.516 (.654)	
EF53. Overreact emotionally				.565 (.707)	
EF59. Easily excitable				.458 (.610)	

(cont.)

TABLE 4.1. *(cont.)*

Factor name/scale items[a]	1	2	3	4	5
EF91. Unable to inhibit showing strong negative or positive emotions				.482 (.657)	
EF92. Have trouble calming myself down once I am emotionally upset				.725 (.825)	
EF93. Cannot seem to regain emotional control and become more reasonable once I am emotional				.732 (.828)	
EF94. Cannot seem to distract myself away from whatever is upsetting me emotionally to help calm me down. I can't refocus my mind to a more positive framework.				.732 (.847)	
EF95. Unable to manage my emotions in order to accomplish my goals successfully or get along well with others				.642 (.786)	
EF96. I remain emotional or upset longer than others				.758 (.829)	
EF97. I find it difficult to walk away from emotionally upsetting encounters with others or leave situations in which I have become very emotional				.711 (.794)	
EF98. I cannot rechannel or redirect my emotions into more positive ways or outlets when I get upset				.699 (.826)	
EF99. I am not able to evaluate an emotionally upsetting event more objectively				.684 (.831)	
EF100. I cannot redefine negative events into more positive viewpoints when I feel strong emotions				.656 (.800)	
5. Self-Motivation					
EF62. Likely to take short cuts in my work and not do all that I am supposed to do					.556 (.632)
EF63. Likely to skip out on work early if my work is boring to do					.569 (.588)
EF64. Do not put as much effort into my work as I should or than others are able to do					.642 (.689)
EF65. Others tell me I am lazy or unmotivated					.641 (.730)
EF66. Have to depend on others to help me get my work done					.608 (.681)
EF67. Things must have an immediate payoff for me or I do not seem to get them done					.555 (.673)
EF68. Have difficulty resisting the urge to do something fun or more interesting when I am supposed to be working					.587 (.648)
EF69. Inconsistent in the quality or quantity of my work performance					.658 (.759)
EF70. Unable to work as well as others without supervision or frequent instruction					.631 (.742)
EF71. I do not have the willpower or determination that others seem to have					.596 (.723)
EF72. I am not able to work toward longer term or delayed rewards as well as others					.612 (.751)
EF73. I cannot resist doing things that produce immediate rewards even if they are not good for me in the long run					.535 (.679)

[a]The number beginning with EF in front of each item reflects the order in which this item appeared on the scale as it was given to the normative sample.
[b]Factor loadings determined via promax rotation are given in parentheses.

Factor 3 accounted for 4.2% of the variance before rotation; it included 18 items from the Self-Restraint (Inhibition) factor of the P-BDEFS, and another item that was rephrased on the BDEFS for clarity. Thus 19 of the eventual 20 items that loaded on this factor were carried forward from the P-BDEFS. There were four items dealing with impulsive emotions on the P-BDEFS that also loaded on this factor in the analysis of that scale. But three of those four items migrated over to the new Self-Regulation of Emotion factor in the analysis of the normative sample. The reason for this shift in factor loadings is obviously the result of our having added new items to this version of the BDEFS that dealt with emotional inhibition and self-regulation, such that a dimension representing this construct of EF now had an opportunity to emerge. The seven highest-loading items on the restructured Self-Restraint factor, in descending order, were these:

- Make impulsive comments to others
- Likely to do things without considering the consequences for doing them
- Fail to consider past relevant events or past personal experiences before responding to situations (I act without thinking)
- Unable to inhibit my reactions or responses to events or others
- Make decisions impulsively
- Don't think about or talk things over with myself before doing something
- Have difficulty stopping my activities or behavior when I should do so

Factor 4, labeled Self-Regulation of Emotion, contained 13 items and accounted for 2.9% of the variance prior to rotation. This factor was the new one that emerged as a result of the addition of items dealing with emotional self-control that were not part of the P-BDEFS, as discussed in Chapter 2. As a result of these new items and the factor they formed, the few items that dealt with impulsive emotion on the P-BDEFS and loaded on the Self-Restraint (Inhibition) factor in our initial research now shifted to having their highest loadings on this new factor. However, even those symptoms ("Overreact emotionally," "Quick to get angry or become upset," "Easily excitable") continued to have their second highest loadings on the Self-Restraint factor, and these were only slightly lower than their loadings on the new Self-Regulation of Emotion factor. Such findings fit with Gross's model of emotional self-control (discussed in Chapter 2), in which a two-stage structure exists: inhibition of strong emotions, followed by efforts at self-regulation of the emotional state. The seven highest-loading items on the Self-Regulation of Emotion factor, in descending order, were as follows:

- I remain emotional or upset longer than others
- Cannot seem to regain emotional control and become more reasonable once I am emotional
- Cannot seem to distract myself away from whatever is upsetting me emotionally to help calm me down. I can't refocus my mind to a more positive framework.
- Have trouble calming myself down once I am emotionally upset
- I find it difficult to walk away from emotionally upsetting encounters with others or leave situations in which I have become very emotional

- I cannot rechannel or redirect my emotions into more positive ways or outlets when I get upset
- I am not able to evaluate an emotionally upsetting event more objectively

Finally, Factor 5 replicated the Self-Motivation factor found in the initial work with the P-BDEFS (see Chapter 2). The factor contained 12 items; 10 of these were carried forward from the P-BDEFS, and the remainder migrated over from the Self-Activation/Concentration factor of the P-BDEFS in this analysis. This factor accounted for 2.5% of the variance prior to rotation. The seven highest-loading items, in descending order, were these:

- Inconsistent in the quality or quantity of my work performance
- Do not put as much effort into my work as I should or than others are able to do
- Others tell me I am lazy or unmotivated
- Unable to work as well as others without supervision or frequent instruction
- I am not able to work toward longer-term or delayed rewards as well as others
- Have to depend on others to help me get my work done
- I do not have the willpower or determination that others seem to have

After the varimax rotation (with Kaiser normalization), the percentages of variance accounted for by the factors, in descending order of variance explained, were as follows:

- Self-Organization/Problem Solving (Factor 1) = 13.6%
- Self-Management to Time (Factor 2) = 11.1%
- Self-Restraint (Factor 3) = 9.2%
- Self-Regulation of Emotion (Factor 4) = 8.9%
- Self-Motivation (Factor 5) = 8.0%

The variances accounted for before and after rotation as shown here are somewhat discrepant from the factor structure and variances explained in the earlier study of the P-BDEFS (see Chapter 2). In that study, the Self-Management to Time factor explained the most variance before and after rotation, and a more robust Self-Activation/Concentration factor was identified. These differences probably arose from the fact that the earlier study was conducted on large samples of adults with ADHD and adults with other clinical disorders who thought they might have ADHD but were not subsequently diagnosed with the disorder. These groups represented more than 65% of the participants in that study, and thus would not be representative of the general population and the difficulties members of this population may report in EF in daily life activities. Although the factor structure in that study was largely the same as that found here for a general population sample, the Self-Activation/Concentration factor scale was not as evident or robust in this analysis as it was in the earlier study. All of this suggests that problems with Self-Management to Time and Self-Activation/Concentration may be far more prominent in adults with ADHD or more closely linked to variation in ADHD symptoms than in a general population sample of adults, as reported here. Perhaps ADHD has a far more detrimental effect on these aspects of EF, and hence the variance that we found associated with these EF factors was greater in the P-BDEFS analysis than was the case in the present analysis. This would certainly be consistent with information suggesting that ADHD is more associated with right prefrontal lobe maldevelopment and dysfunctioning, and with deficits in self-awareness across time, nonverbal working memory, and inhibitory tasks (all of which are more likely to be lateralized to the right prefrontal region).

Scale Construction

The items in Table 4.1 were used to create the subscales for the BDEFS published here. Most items were kept in their original sequence on the scale, just as they were presented to the normative sample during the survey. We did this because item organization can influence symptom endorsements by respondents (Mitchell, Knouse, Nelson-Gray, & Kwapil, 2009), and so items needed to remain as close to their original sequence in the norming process as possible, so as not to reduce the applicability of the norms for the final scale. But some items had to be moved from their locations in the original sequence because the results of the PCFA showed that they should actually be assigned to a different factor than the one to which they were originally thought to belong. For ease of scoring the BDEFS, the items were reorganized in their positions so that all items pertaining to a single factor were located in the same section of the scale. This sequence was largely that presented to the normative sample. Because the items for Self-Management to Time appeared first in this sequence, they were kept in that order, followed by the items for Self-Organization/Problem Solving, then the items for Self-Restraint, followed by the items for Self-Motivation, and concluding with the section containing the items for Self-Regulation of Emotion. Therefore, five subscale sections presently exist on the BDEFS. This makes scoring the scale easier, as the examiner can simply sum the scores for the items in each section (subscale) to compute that subscale's score. These subscale total scores can then be summed to compute the Total EF Summary Score (see Chapter 8 for detailed scoring instructions).

The final 89 items that were used to create the BDEFS Long Form (BDEFS-LF) were then resubmitted to PCFA with varimax rotation, which yielded the same five factors and the same item assignments to factors as in the original analysis. The five factors explained 53.2% of the variance. The explained percentages of variance for these factors after rotation were as follows:

- Self-Organization/Problem Solving (Factor 1) = 13.9%
- Self-Management to Time (Factor 2) = 12.0%
- Self-Regulation of Emotion (Factor 3) = 10.2%
- Self-Restraint (Factor 4) = 9.0%
- Self-Motivation (Factor 5) = 8.1%

Creation of the ADHD-EF Index

Our previous research using the P-BDEFS indicated that adult ADHD is associated with significant impairment in EF in daily life activities in the majority of adults with the disorder (Barkley & Murphy, 2010b). The database from that earlier research study was therefore used here to identify those items from the P-BDEFS that were most likely to identify the adults clinically diagnosed with ADHD, relative to the Community control group. The results of a binary logistic regression showed that just five items were needed to classify these two groups with 98.1% overall accuracy (99.1% of cases with ADHD and 96.9% of Community cases). The same form of analysis was then used to compare the ADHD group with the Clinical control group in that study, consisting of adults who thought they had ADHD but subsequently were found not to meet *Diagnostic and Statistical Manual of Mental Disorders*, fourth edition (DSM-IV; American Psychiatric Association, 2000), criteria. This time, seven items best discriminated the groups, with an accuracy of 82.9% for the ADHD group but just 56% for the Clinical group and an overall classification rate of 72.3%. This means that discriminating patients with ADHD from other clinical patients having other disorders is not as easily done with rating scale items alone. One of the items out of these seven was also found in the initial analysis above comparing the ADHD and Community groups. These two sets of items were combined to create a brief index based on these 11 most discriminating items for adult ADHD classification. These items were as follows:

- Procrastinate or put off doing things until the last minute
- Have trouble planning ahead or preparing for upcoming events
- Have difficulty motivating myself to stick with my work and get it done
- Have trouble completing one activity before starting into a new one
- I have trouble organizing my thoughts
- Have difficulty stopping my activities or behavior when I should do so
- Have difficulty changing my behavior when I am given feedback about my mistakes
- Not aware of things I say or do
- More likely to drive a motor vehicle much faster than others (Excessive speeding)
- Likely to take short cuts in my work and not do all that I am supposed to do
- Have to depend on others to help me get my work done

These 11 items therefore constitute the ADHD-EF Index, which can suggest to an examiner that a person may be at risk for having adult ADHD and may need to be evaluated further. The Index items are indicated on the two BDEFS-LF forms in the Appendix by shaded boxes on their item numbers.

Creation of the BDEFS Short Form

There may be situations in which an examiner or respondent does not have time to complete the 89-item BDEFS-LF. In such cases, a quick screening tool for assessing the possibility of deficits in EF in daily life may be desirable. The BDEFS Short Form (BDEFS-SF) was created to serve this purpose. It is composed of the four highest-loading items from each of the five subscales, and thus provides a 20-item EF screener. Both a self-report form and a report form for another adult to complete about a person are provided for both the BDEFS-LF and BDEFS-SF. All these forms can be found in the Appendix. A separate score sheet was created just for the BDEFS-SF, apart from those used to score the BDEFS-LF. Information on the reliability and validity of both the BDEFS-LF and BDEFS-SF is provided in later chapters.

Frequency of Item Responses

It is clinically and scientifically informative to examine the percentage of respondents in the normative sample who endorsed each of the item responses. This information can suggest how common or uncommon such symptoms of EF deficits in daily life activities are likely to be. Neuropsychologists, for example, may want to know the proportion of the population that endorses particular types of EF symptoms at various relative frequency estimates. The information can also be used to determine what frequency of occurrence for each item can be used to indicate that this item at this frequency level can be judged to be a symptom of an actual deficit, rather than a common occurrence in the population. For instance, if the vast majority of adults answer an item with "never or rarely" or "sometimes," then responses of "often" or "very often" can be considered to indicate a symptom of an EF deficit.

A "symptom" in this case would be defined as a behavioral complaint occurring at a frequency that is relatively low in the population and so may be indicative of disorder. Whether it is or not, of course, is eventually a question of validity to be tested against other forms of information. To gain some idea about how often typical adults endorse items of EF problems in daily life and at what frequency of occurrence (never or rarely, sometimes, often, very often), the percentage of adults in the normative sample who endorsed each of the possible answers to each item was computed. The results appear in Table 4.2. What this table clearly shows is that for the vast majority of items, with a few exceptions, the vast majority of this general population sample endorsed most items at a frequency of either "never or rarely" or "sometimes." Answers of "often" and especially "very often" appeared to occur in less than 1–10% of the population in most cases (though clearly there were a few exceptions). But if one wanted to identify a symptom of EF, it does not seem at all unreasonable to use an answer of "often" or "very often" to indicate the possibility of symptom status. The examiner should therefore not just focus on scoring the BDEFS through simple summation of items, but should inspect the scale for items on each subscale that were endorsed with responses of 3 (often) or 4 (very often). This can provide another perspective on just how symptomatic a respondent may be in each component of EF assessed by each subscale.

The next chapter describes the relationship of BDEFS scores to various demographic and other factors in the normative sample. These issues pertain to the question of how best to present the norms provided in this manual for purposes of scoring both the BDEFS-LF and the BDEFS-SF.

TABLE 4.2. Percentage of the Normative Sample That Endorsed Each Possible Answer to Each Item on the BDEFS

	Never or rarely	Sometimes	Often	Very often
Self-Management to Time items				
1. Procrastinate or put off doing things until the last minute	21.5	50.0	19.9	8.6
2. Poor sense of time	53.6	36.0	7.9	2.4
3. Waste or mismanage my time	27.1	54.9	13.5	4.6
4. Not prepared on time for work or assigned tasks	70.7	23.2	4.6	1.4
5. Fail to meet deadlines for assignments	77.7	18.7	2.6	1.0
6. Have trouble planning ahead or preparing for upcoming events	58.6	35.9	4.2	1.3
7. Forget to do things I am supposed to do	38.4	50.4	8.6	2.7
8. Can't seem to accomplish the goals I set for myself	40.3	46.0	10.6	3.0
9. Late for work or scheduled appointments	78.9	16.0	3.6	1.5
10. Can't seem to hold in mind things I need to remember to do	44.1	43.7	9.3	2.9
11. Can't seem to get things done unless there is an immediate deadline	46.3	38.8	11.2	3.7
12. Have difficulty judging how much time it will take to do something or get somewhere	55.6	35.2	7.3	1.9
13. Have trouble motivating myself to start work	36.6	45.3	13.0	5.1
14. Have difficulty motivating myself to stick with my work and get it done	51.1	35.4	9.4	4.1
15. Not motivated to prepare in advance for things I know I am supposed to do	51.2	38.5	7.8	2.5
16. Have trouble completing one activity before starting into a new one	43.0	42.8	10.2	4.1
17. Have trouble doing what I tell myself to do	46.8	40.9	9.9	2.3
18. Difficulties following through on promises or commitments I may make to others	74.2	21.5	3.2	1.0
19. Lack self-discipline	46.9	42.1	7.7	3.3
20. Have difficulty arranging or doing my work by its priority or importance; can't "prioritize" well	64.6	29.1	5.1	1.2
21. Find it hard to get started or get going on things I need to get done	45.3	41.6	9.4	3.7
Self-Organization/Problem Solving items				
22. I do not seem to anticipate the future as much or as well as others	59.6	33.7	5.0	1.0
23. Can't seem to remember what I previously heard or read about	41.6	46.8	9.0	2.6
24. I have trouble organizing my thoughts	55.4	36.7	6.4	1.4
25. When I am shown something complicated to do, I cannot keep the information in mind so as to imitate or do it correctly	53.4	38.4	6.8	1.4
26. I have trouble considering various options for doing things and weighing their consequences	68.0	26.5	4.1	1.4
27. Have difficulties saying what I want to say	49.6	38.2	9.8	2.4
28. Unable to come up with or invent as many solutions to problems as others seem to do	60.3	33.2	4.9	1.6
29. Find myself at a loss for words when I want to explain something to others	51.5	38.3	7.6	2.6
30. Have trouble putting my thoughts down in writing as well or as quickly as others	58.6	30.4	8.4	2.6
31. Feel I am not as creative or inventive as others of my level of intelligence	52.2	37.3	7.8	2.7
32. In trying to accomplish goals or assignments, I find I am not able to think of as many ways of doing things as others	58.3	34.4	5.6	1.7

(cont.)

TABLE 4.2. *(cont.)*

	Never or rarely	Sometimes	Often	Very often
33. Have trouble learning new or complex activities as well as others	57.5	35.3	5.5	1.7
34. Have difficulty explaining things in their proper order or sequence	64.3	29.1	4.8	1.8
35. Can't seem to get to the point of my explanations as quickly as others	53.8	37.3	7.0	1.8
36. Have trouble doing things in their proper order or sequence	71.5	24.7	2.9	1.0
37. Unable to "think on my feet" or respond as effectively as others to unexpected events	60.7	30.3	6.6	2.4
38. I am slower than others at solving problems I encounter in my daily life	69.2	24.7	4.3	1.8
39. Easily distracted by irrelevant events or thoughts when I must concentrate on something	48.2	41.5	8.0	2.3
40. Not able to comprehend what I read as well as I should be able to do; have to reread material to get its meaning	51.1	36.9	9.0	3.0
41. Cannot focus my attention on tasks or work as well as others	69.3	25.3	3.8	1.6
42. Easily confused	71.7	23.5	3.3	1.5
43. Can't seem to sustain my concentration on reading, paperwork, lectures, or work	60.0	30.5	7.2	2.2
44. Find it hard to focus on what is important from what is not important when I do things	71.8	23.7	3.0	1.5
45. I don't seem to process information as quickly or as accurately as others	66.5	28.0	3.4	2.0
Self-Restraint items				
46. Find it difficult to tolerate waiting; impatient	32.5	43.7	17.5	6.3
47. Make decisions impulsively	44.4	45.6	8.2	1.8
48. Unable to inhibit my reactions or responses to events or others	54.0	37.1	7.4	1.5
49. Have difficulty stopping my activities or behavior when I should do so	58.9	33.5	5.4	2.2
50. Have difficulty changing my behavior when I am given feedback about my mistakes	58.1	35.6	5.0	1.2
51. Make impulsive comments to others	50.9	39.7	7.4	2.0
52. Likely to do things without considering the consequences for doing them	69.7	25.9	3.4	1.0
53. Change my plans at the last minute on a whim or last minute impulse	57.5	36.2	4.7	1.6
54. Fail to consider past relevant events or past personal experiences before responding to situations (I act without thinking)	68.0	28.4	2.4	1.2
55. Not aware of things I say or do	76.0	20.6	2.4	1.0
56. Have difficulty being objective about things that affect me	54.1	38.5	6.5	0.9
57. Find it hard to take other people's perspectives about a problem or situation	56.5	37.3	5.1	1.0
58. Don't think about or talk things over with myself before doing something	63.3	31.3	4.5	0.9
59. Trouble following the rules in a situation	74.9	21.5	2.9	0.6
60. More likely to drive a motor vehicle much faster than others (Excessive speeding)	70.0	22.4	5.5	2.1
61. Have a low tolerance for frustrating situations	39.1	44.2	13.1	3.7
62. Cannot inhibit my emotions as well as others	59.6	31.8	7.0	1.6

(cont.)

TABLE 4.2. *(cont.)*

	Never or rarely	Sometimes	Often	Very often
63. I don't look ahead and think about what the future outcomes will be before I do something (I don't use my foresight)	69.9	25.1	3.6	1.4
64. I engage in risk taking activities more than others are likely to do	74.1	21.1	3.6	1.3
Self-Motivation items				
65. Likely to take short cuts in my work and not do all that I am supposed to do	70.3	25.3	3.4	1.0
66. Likely to skip out on work early if my work is boring to do	78.9	17.4	2.9	0.8
67. Do not put as much effort into my work as I should or than others are able to do	77.6	18.4	3.3	0.7
68. Others tell me I am lazy or unmotivated	86.9	9.9	2.2	1.0
69. Have to depend on others to help me get my work done	84.7	12.8	1.4	1.0
70. Things must have an immediate payoff for me or I do not seem to get them done	73.7	23.1	2.3	0.9
71. Have difficulty resisting the urge to do something fun or more interesting when I am supposed to be working	64.5	28.8	4.6	2.1
72. Inconsistent in the quality or quantity of my work performance	80.9	16.0	2.2	0.9
73. Unable to work as well as others without supervision or frequent instruction	89.2	7.7	2.2	0.9
74. I do not have the willpower or determination that others seem to have	72.8	21.5	3.8	1.9
75. I am not able to work toward longer term or delayed rewards as well as others	76.6	18.3	3.4	1.7
76. I cannot resist doing things that produce immediate rewards even if they are not good for me in the long run	70.5	24.7	3.4	1.4
Self-Regulation of Emotion items				
77. Quick to get angry or become upset	48.8	38.8	9.4	3.0
78. Overreact emotionally	49.0	40.4	8.6	2.0
79. Easily excitable	53.5	37.0	7.5	2.0
80. Unable to inhibit showing strong negative or positive emotions	57.2	34.9	5.9	2.0
81. Have trouble calming myself down once I am emotionally upset	54.9	34.7	7.5	2.9
82. Cannot seem to regain emotional control and become more reasonable once I am emotional	70.1	23.4	4.4	2.2
83. Cannot seem to distract myself away from whatever is upsetting me emotionally to help calm me down. I can't refocus my mind to a more positive framework.	60.8	30.2	6.7	2.2
84. Unable to manage my emotions in order to accomplish my goals successfully or get along well with others	77.4	17.9	3.3	1.4
85. I remain emotional or upset longer than others	66.4	25.4	6.0	2.2
86. I find it difficult to walk away from emotionally upsetting encounters with others or leave situations in which I have become very emotional	67.1	26.2	4.6	2.2
87. I cannot rechannel or redirect my emotions into more positive ways or outlets when I get upset	64.1	28.9	5.1	1.8
88. I am not able to evaluate an emotionally upsetting event more objectively	66.5	28.3	4.0	1.2
89. I cannot redefine negative events into more positive viewpoints when I feel strong emotions	59.7	32.7	5.6	2.0

Note. Items are arranged in the order in which they appear in the final scale. See the BDEFS-LF: Self-Report in the Appendix.

CHAPTER 5

Relationship of BDEFS Scores to Demographic Factors in the Normative Sample

This chapter describes the relationship of various demographic factors to the BDEFS subscale scores and Total EF Summary Score for the entire sample of 1,249 adults. (All references to the BDEFS are to the BDEFS-LF, except in the discussion of the BDEFS-LF and BDEFS-SF score sheets at the end of the chapter.)

Age

Age was not found to correlate significantly with the Self-Organization/Problem Solving subscale ($r = .019$, $p =$ NS). But age was observed to correlate to a small but significant degree with the remaining five BDEFS scores: Self-Management to Time ($r = -.13$, $p < .001$); Self-Restraint ($r = -.08$, $p = .007$); Self-Regulation of Emotion ($r = -.11$, $p < .001$); Self-Motivation ($r = -.13$, $p < .001$); and Total EF Summary Score ($r = -.09$, $p = .002$). This had also been true of the P-BDEFS in the UMASS Study of adults with ADHD, a Clinical control group, and a Community control group. In the UMASS Study, three of the five self-rated subscales showed a low but significant correlation with participant age: Self-Management to Time ($r = -.11$, $p = .05$); Self-Motivation ($r = -.21$, $p < .001$); and Self-Activation/Concentration ($r = -.11$, $p = .04$). This was true for these same three subscales rated by others: Self-Management to Time ($r = -.16$, $p = .01$); Self-Motivation ($r = -.27$, $p < .001$); and Self-Activation/Concentration ($r = -.16$, $p = .009$). Difficulties with EF in daily life activities thus appear to be somewhat more common in younger than in middle-aged or older adults.

Correlation analyses, however, can disguise nonlinear effects within such data, particularly when there is good reason to believe that EF problems may decline with age but then increase in late life. We therefore also analyzed the relationship of age to the BDEFS scores, using seven age groupings (18–29, 30–39, 40–49, 50–59, 60–69, 70–79, and 80+ years) in an analysis of variance. The effect of age was significant for five of the BDEFS scores and marginally so for Self-Restraint. The results were as follows: Self-Organization/Problem Solving ($F = 2.15$, $p = .045$); Self-Management to Time ($F = 4.17$, $p < .001$); Self-Restraint ($F = 2.02$, $p = .061$); Self-Regulation of Emotion ($F = 3.32$, $p = .003$); Self-Motivation ($F = 3.73$, $p = .001$); and Total EF Summary Score ($F = 2.49$, $p = .021$). But the pattern of these mean scores proves the point made above about the possibility of nonlinear effects—in this case, an apparent curvilinear relationship in the data.

The mean score for each of these seven age groups for the BDEFS Total EF Summary Score is shown in Figure 5.1. It suggests a slight decline in this score with age, yet with a slight increase at ages 50–59 followed by a decline in the next two age groups, and then a rise in the score after age 80 years (this last finding is not surprising). The individual BDEFS subscale scores for each age group are shown in Figure 5.2. Again, visual inspection suggests a general small decline in the different domains of EF in daily life activities with age. But there is a slight upturn of some subscales at ages 50–59 before the mild downward decline in EF problems continues into the next later two age groups. Then there is an apparent rise in some subscales after 80 years of age. The numerical differences across the age groups, however, are quite small relative to the mean scores at each level. They reflect no more than a 1- or 2-point change in scores with age group for each of the subscale scores and a 5- to 11-point change for the Total EF Summary Score. This suggests about a

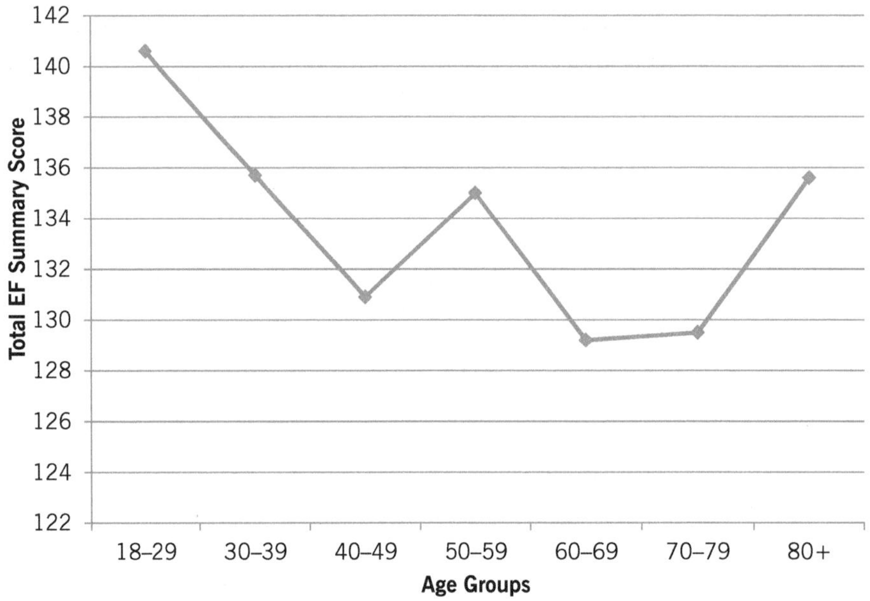

FIGURE 5.1. Total EF Summary Score for each of seven age groups: 18–29, 30–39, 40–49, 50–59, 60–69, 70–79, and 80+ years.

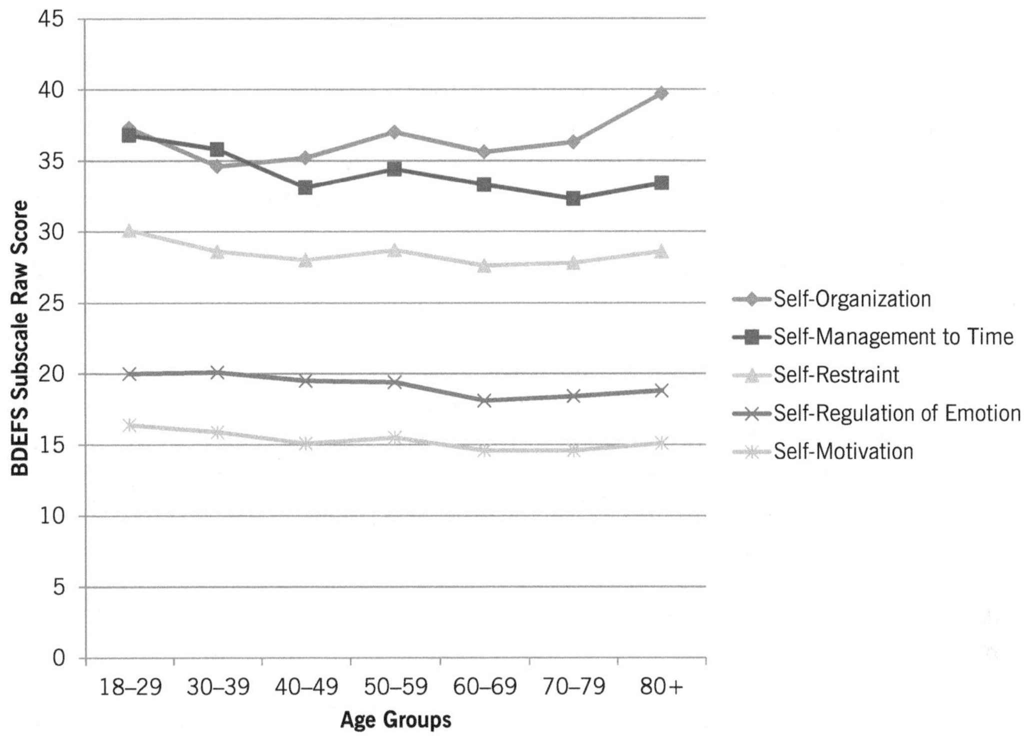

FIGURE 5.2. Specific BDEFS subscale scores for each of seven age groups: 18–29, 30–39, 40–49, 50–59, 60–69, 70–79, and 80+ years.

10% decline in mean scores across the age span examined here until age 80 in the severity of EF deficits in daily life activities. Although not identical to these results, a similar age-related decline was evident in the normative sample for another rating scale of EF in adults, the BRIEF (Roth et al., 2005).

It is possible that the pattern here reflects a true decline in the occurrence of EF problems with age until late life, when such problems begin to increase slightly. After all, the PFC is believed not to attain its final maturation until the late 20s to early 30s, and so finding somewhat more EF deficits in the youngest age group makes sense. But these changes may also reflect a decline with age in the willingness to participate in survey research among those having higher EF problems, such that only those with fewer EF problems are willing to participate in such research, at least until late life.

Another reasonable explanation may be that this decline reflects the differential survival of those with fewer EF deficits relative to individuals with greater deficits, who may experience a shorter life expectancy. Past research has shown that EF deficits are related to impairment in various major life activities (Barkley & Fischer, in press; Barkley & Murphy, 2010a). Also, EF may well be related to the personality trait of conscientiousness, such that deficits in EF are associated with lower levels of this personality trait. Research has shown that individuals placing in the lowest quartile of conscientiousness have a shorter life expectancy by an average of 7 years than do those with higher levels of this trait (Friedman et al., 1995). This may also be the case for persons with ADHD, given the growing health risks (e.g., smoking, alcoholism, drug use and abuse, risk for accidental injuries, and risk for coronary heart disease) documented to date in relation to this disorder (Barkley et al., 2008). As already noted, ADHD is closely associated with deficits in EF in daily activities. It is therefore not merely conjectural that individuals with greater EF problems are likely to have a shorter life expectancy, and thus not as likely to be represented in population surveys of older adults.

Pairwise comparisons indicated that where age groups differed, it was principally that the 18- to 29-year-olds differed from the remainder of the age groups. On some scales, the 80+-year-olds also began to differ significantly from the other groups, in that an increase in EF problems appeared to be occurring at this age. Inspection of all of the results for age, along with the distributions for the scores on each scale, indicated that four large age groupings could be created from the initial seven discussed above. These groupings appeared to be sensible, given the changes that may well occur with age on EF. Yet they allowed the creation of relatively equal yet substantial sample sizes within each age grouping, to maximize the representativeness of the norms for each age group. Only 31 participants were 82 years of age or older. Given that this older age group appeared to be demonstrating an increase in some types of EF problems, we dropped these participants from further consideration. In any case, this group was far too small to provide adequate norms of the U.S. population in this age range (82+). Thus the BDEFS normative information on the score sheets in the Appendix is appropriate for individuals between 18 and 81 years of age. The final four age groupings were 18–34, 35–49, 50–64, and 65–81

TABLE 5.1. BDEFS Results for Each of Four Age Groups

	Age groups										
	(1) 18–34		(2) 35–49		(3) 50–64		(4) 65–81				
Score	Mean	*SD*	Mean	*SD*	Mean	*SD*	Mean	*SD*	*F*	*p*	Contrasts
Self-Organize	36.7	12.3	34.7	12.6	36.6	12.2	36.1	9.6	1.84	NS	1 > 2 2 > 3
Time Mgmt.	36.7	11.8	33.7	11.5	34.4	10.7	32.2	8.1	9.23	< .001	1 > 2,3,4 3 > 4
Self-Restraint	30.0	9.6	27.8	9.1	28.6	7.9	27.4	6.6	5.21	.003	1 > 2,3,4
Emotion Reg.	20.5	8.0	19.7	8.0	19.0	6.3	18.2	5.2	5.84	.001	1 > 3,4 2 > 4
Self-Motivate	16.5	5.8	15.2	5.2	15.3	4.8	14.4	3.1	9.03	< .001	1 > 2,3,4 3 > 4
EF Summary	140.4	40.0	131.1	40.3	133.9	36.0	128.3	26.3	6.04	< .001	1 > 2,3,4

Note. Self-Organize, Self-Organization/Problem Solving subscale; Time Mgmt., Self-Management to Time subscale; Emotion Reg., Self-Regulation of Emotion subscale; Self-Motivate, Self-Motivation subscale; EF Summary, Total EF Summary Score; *F*, results for the *F*-test from the analysis of variance; *p*, probability value for the *F*-test if ≤ .05; NS, not significant. Contrasts are the results of the pairwise comparisons of the four age groups.

years. These yielded sample sizes per age grouping of 305, 316, 322, and 275, respectively, for a total sample of 1,218. The results for the comparisons among the age groups are shown in Table 5.1.

Sex

A comparison of the 620 males with the 619 females from the entire original sample indicated no significant differences on Self-Organization/Problem Solving, Self-Management to Time, and the Total EF Summary Scores. However, men reported having marginally higher problem scores on Self-Restraint ($p = .055$) and significantly greater problems on Self-Motivation ($p < .05$) than women. In contrast, women reported having higher problem scores on Self-Regulation of Emotion ($p < .05$) than men; a similar result was observed in the normative data for the adult version of the BRIEF (Roth et al., 2005). The results for these analyses are shown in Table 5.2. Though significant sex differences emerged on Self-Regulation of Emotion and Self-Motivation, the differences in mean scores for those two subscales were relatively small. The distributions of scores were then examined, and while scores within the average range were typically equivalent between men and women on most subscales, the differences between the sexes became more evident as the scores became more extreme. The results thus suggest that norms for men and women should be presented separately for scoring the BDEFS. Although similar results for sex differences were evident on the adult version of the BRIEF, those developers elected not to portray their norms separately for each sex (Roth et al., 2005).

Using the entire sample, the next analysis examined whether there was an interaction of age with sex on any of the BDEFS scores. Main effects for these two variables have already been discussed above and so are ignored here. Two-way analysis of variance was used to examine this issue. The findings are portrayed in Figures 5.3–5.8 for each of the BDEFS subscales and the Total EF Summary Score.

(text resumes on page 61)

TABLE 5.2. Comparison of Males and Females on BDEFS Scores

	Men		Women			
Score	Mean	*SD*	Mean	*SD*	*F*	*p*
Self-Organize	35.7	12.3	36.5	11.3	1.55	NS
Time Mgmt.	34.4	11.3	34.2	10.3	0.12	NS
Self-Restraint	29.0	9.0	28.0	7.8	3.70	.055
Emotion Reg.	19.0	7.2	19.8	6.9	3.91	.048
Self-Motivate	15.9	5.4	14.9	4.3	13.80	< .001
EF Summary	133.9	38.8	133.4	34.2	0.07	NS

Note. See footnote to Table 5.1 for explanations.

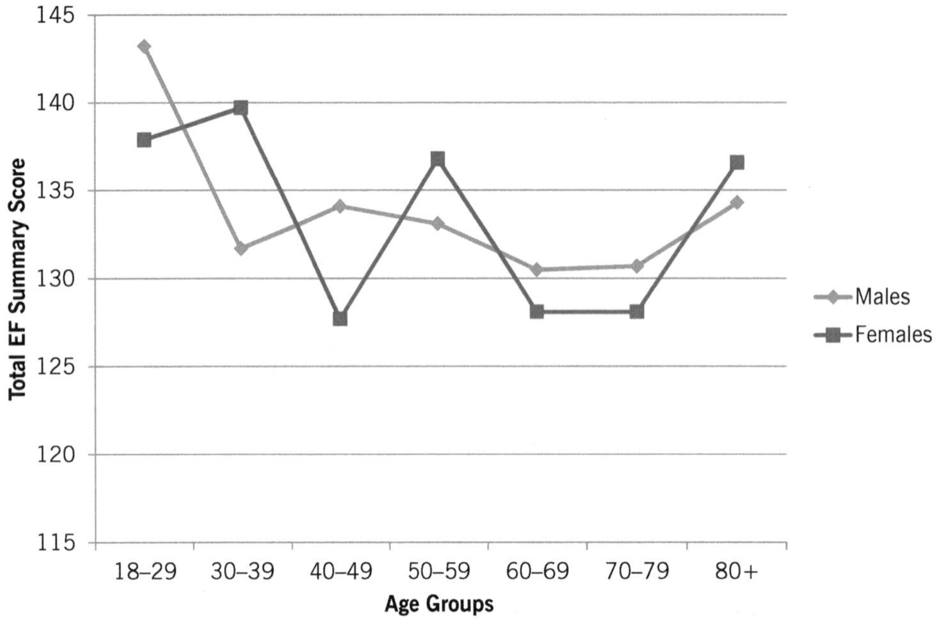

FIGURE 5.3. Total EF Summary Score for each sex within each of seven age groups: 18–29, 30–39, 40–49, 50–59, 60–69, 70–79, and 80+ years.

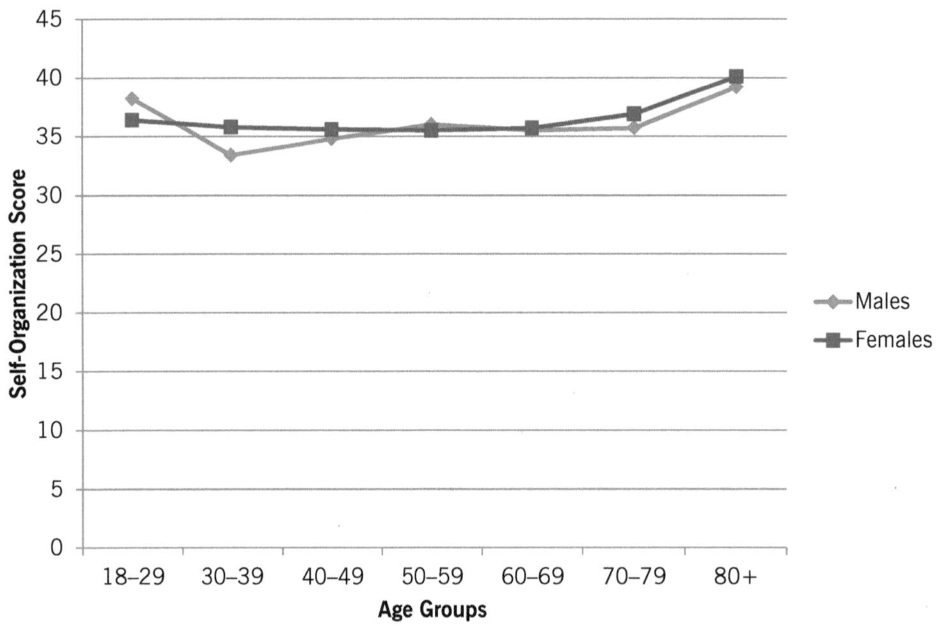

FIGURE 5.4. Self-Organization/Problem Solving subscale score for each sex within each of seven age groups: 18–29, 30–39, 40–49, 50–59, 60–69, 70–79, and 80+ years.

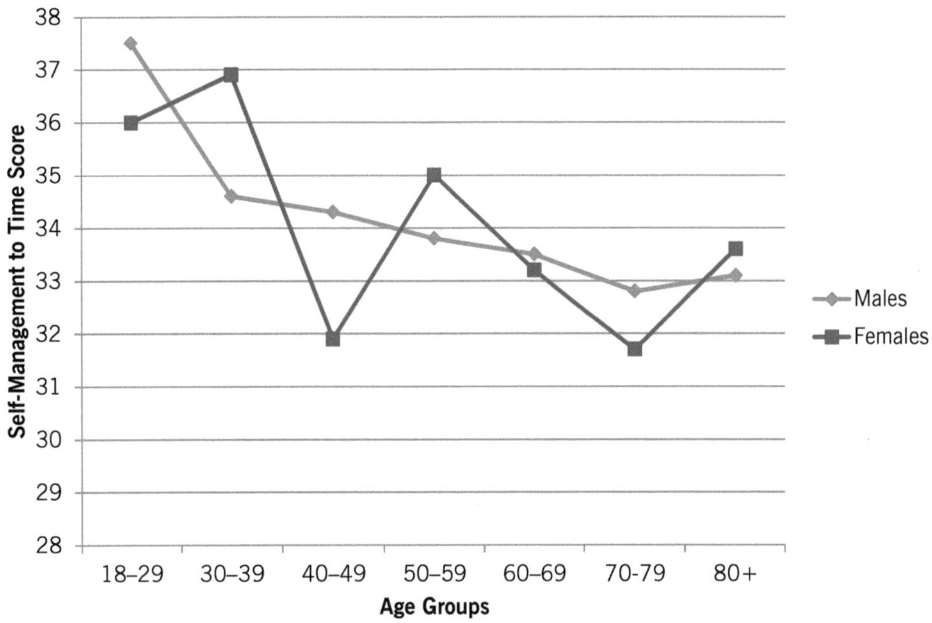

FIGURE 5.5. Self-Management to Time subscale score for each sex within each of seven age groups: 18–29, 30–39, 40–49, 50–59, 60–69, 70–79, and 80+ years.

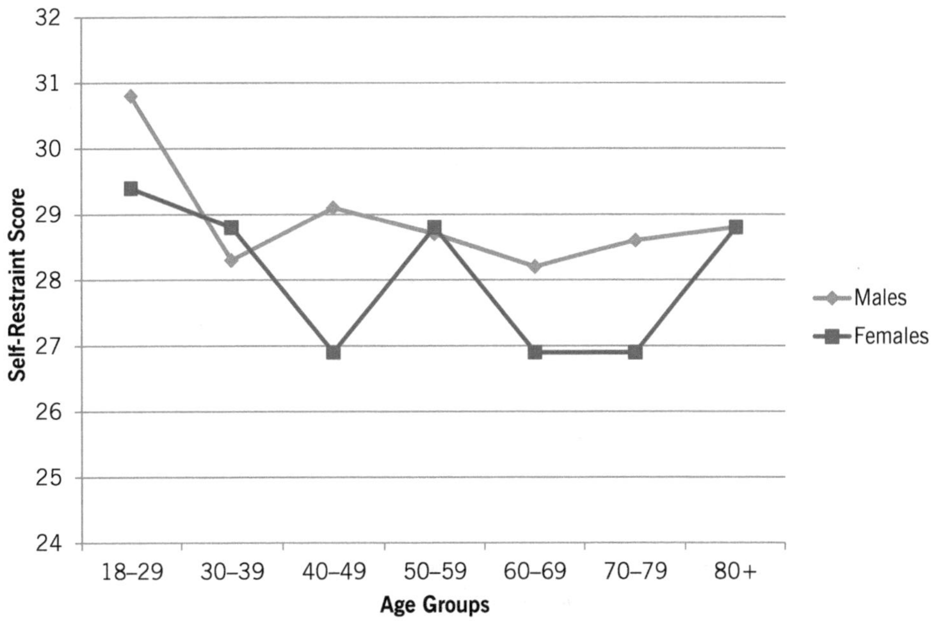

FIGURE 5.6. Self-Restraint subscale score for each sex within each of seven age groups: 18–29, 30–39, 40–49, 50–59, 60–69, 70–79, and 80+ years.

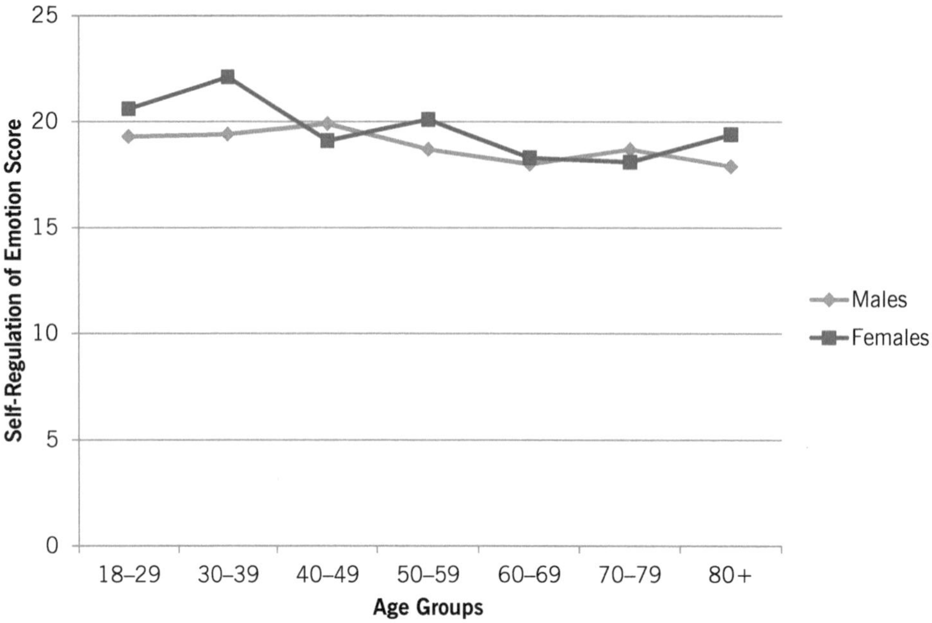

FIGURE 5.7. Self-Regulation of Emotion subscale score for each sex within each of seven age groups: 18–29, 30–39, 40–49, 50–59, 60–69, 70–79, and 80+ years.

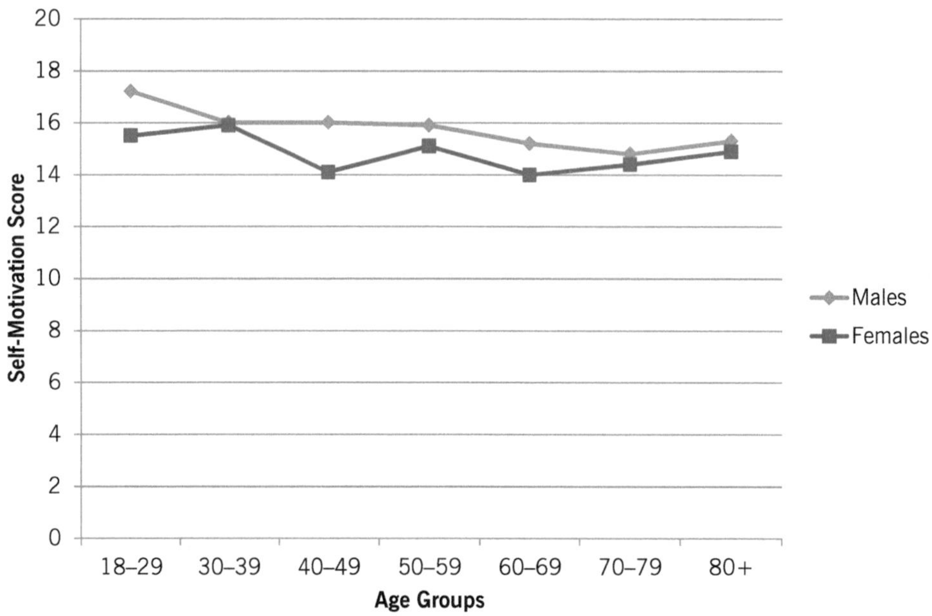

FIGURE 5.8. Self-Motivation subscale score for each sex within each of seven age groups: 18–29, 30–39, 40–49, 50–59, 60–69, 70–79, and 80+ years.

Results indicated that there were no significant interactions on any of the subscales or on the Total EF Summary Score between sex and age grouping, nor did any analyses even approach significance ($p < .05$). But the pattern of results may help to explain why an overall increase in the Total EF Summary Score occurred at ages 50–59 in the results discussed above and shown in Figure 5.1. There appears to be a steeper decrease in EF problems on some subscales in females than in males, but a slight increase in females at ages 50–59 before declining again until late life (age 80+). In other words, the change in women's reports of EF problems at ages 50–59 is what accounts for the increase at this age in some EF problems (i.e., time management). An interesting question to be explored in future research is whether this change in EF problems corresponds to the onset of perimenopause and the frequent complaints of women at this time concerning its adverse effect on working memory (i.e., forgetfulness).

To determine whether the norms should be displayed for each sex within each of the final four age groups we created (18–34, 35–49, 50–64, 65–81), we examined the distribution of BDEFS scores for each sex within each age group. Here we were trying to determine whether the scores associated with the various percentile scores actually differed enough between the sexes to warrant displaying such percentile cutoff scores separately by sex. After all, the mean score differences noted in Table 5.2 between men and women were exceptionally small, probably reaching statistical significance mainly because of the large sample size being evaluated here. The inspections suggested that the score differences, though small, were sufficiently different (especially at the extreme upper end of the distributions) to warrant displaying the percentile scores for each sex within each of these four age groups. But the percentile scores for the entire sample within each age group are also presented. Those scores are likely to be the most reliable, as they are based on twice the sample size for each age group than is the case for each sex displayed separately. It is recommended that clinicians score the scale both ways—initially making sex-based comparisons within an individual's age group, and then comparing the individual to the entire age group with both sexes combined.

Ethnic Group

The next issue to address in considering how best to portray the norms for scoring purposes was whether there existed any significant relationship of ethnic group to the BDEFS scores. One-way analysis of variance revealed no significant effects of ethnic group on four of the five BDEFS subscale scores or on the Total EF Summary Score. But there was a significant effect on the Self-Motivation subscale ($F = 3.03$, $df = 4/1{,}234$, $p = .017$). Pairwise comparisons indicated that Hispanic participants ($M = 16.8$, $SD = 6.7$) reported somewhat higher levels of problems with this area of EF than did white participants ($M = 15.2$, $SD = 4.6$) or those categorized as other non-Hispanic (mostly Asian) ($M = 14.8$, $SD = 3.9$). Participants of black ethnicity ($M = 15.7$, $SD = 5.0$) did not differ from any of the other groups, nor did those individuals classified as identifying with two or more ethnic categories ($M = 15.9$, $SD = 7.0$). Consequently, there seems to be little or no clinical value in displaying the norms for each ethnic group for scoring of the BDEFS.

Geographic Region

It also seemed important to determine whether there existed any geographic regional differences in the BDEFS scores that might have importance for the interpretation of the norms. An analysis of variance using the entire normative sample (*N* = 1,249) was conducted to compare results for the four major U.S. regions. The results are shown in Table 5.3. There were no significant differences for any of the subscales or for the Total EF Summary Score, nor did any of the comparisons even approach significance. It is therefore possible to collapse the geographic regions together for purposes of displaying the normative information on this sample.

Creation of the BDEFS-LF and BDEFS-SF Score Sheets

BDEFS-LF Score Sheets

Raw Score Totals

Two forms (Self-Report, Other-Report) are provided in the Appendix for the BDEFS-LF. A total of 12 score sheets—one for each gender within each of the four age groups (ages 18–34, 35–49, 50–64, and 65–81), and one for each age group with the genders combined—have been created for scoring and interpreting the BDEFS-LF: Self-Report only. No norms were collected for the Other-Report. The norms presented on each of the score sheets are set forth separately for each of the five BDEFS-LF subscale total raw scores, the Total EF Summary Score, and the ADHD-EF Index. These are the final sample sizes on which these score sheets are based:

- Ages 18–29 (*n* = 305; males = 151, females = 154)
- Ages 30–44 (*n* = 316; males = 159, females = 157)
- Ages 45–64 (*n* = 322; males = 161, females = 161)
- Ages 65–81 (*n* = 275; males = 138, females = 137)

TABLE 5.3. BDEFS Results for Each of Four U.S. Geographical Regions

	Regions									
	Northeast		Midwest		South		West			
Score	Mean	*SD*	Mean	*SD*	Mean	*SD*	Mean	*SD*	*F*	*p*
Self-Organize	35.0	11.5	36.3	12.0	35.9	11.9	37.3	11.5	1.59	NS
Time Mgmt.	33.4	10.2	33.5	10.5	34.8	11.3	35.1	10.5	1.92	NS
Self-Restraint	28.4	8.4	28.1	8.3	28.7	8.7	28.7	8.2	0.38	NS
Emotion Reg.	19.1	6.7	19.4	6.9	19.4	7.4	19.4	6.8	0.15	NS
Self-Motivate	15.0	4.4	15.2	5.1	15.4	4.7	15.7	5.4	0.98	NS
EF Summary	130.9	35.2	132.6	37.3	134.3	36.9	136.2	36.1	1.02	NS

Note. See footnote to Table 5.1 for explanations.

The means and standard deviations for the five subscales and the Total EF Summary Score by sex within each of these four age groupings for the BDEFS-LF are shown in Table 5.4. These distributions were used to create the score sheets that appear in the Appendix. The percentiles for the combined samples (men and women) are likely to be the most valid or indicative of the population in that age group as a whole. Raw score ranges are presented for the 1st–25th, 26th–50th, and 51st–75th percentiles. This is done to save space and because the specific percentiles associated with lower scores on the BDEFS are of limited clinical value beyond the information provided by these three ranges. It is only above the 75th percentile that the specific percentiles become more useful for clinical purposes.

EF Symptom Count

As indicated in Chapter 4, it is reasonable to consider an item answered as 3 (often) or 4 (very often) to be a symptom of deficient EF, given the relatively low frequency with which items were answered in this way (see Table 4.2). It would seem to be of some clinical interest to know how many BDEFS items were answered in this fashion by the normative sample. This score was computed, and the results are graphically depicted in Figure 5.9. The EF Symptom Count is portrayed by age group only because there was no significant sex difference in this score, nor was there a significant interaction of age with sex; there was, however, a significant effect of age grouping on these results. The specific results appear in Table 5.4. In general, there was a linear decline in symptom counts with age. The 18- to 34-year-old group endorsed significantly more symptoms than the other three groups. The 35- to 49-year-olds and the 50- to 64-year-olds also reported more symptoms than the 65- to 81-year-olds. Using these results, we devised a separate score sheet for the EF Symptom Count, and the normative sample was used to specify the symptom counts that were equivalent to the ≤ 50th, 51st–75th, and (individually) ≥ 76th and higher percentiles for each age group. Again, specific percentile breakdown scores are provided only above the 75th percentile, given the limited clinical value associated with lower symptom counts.

BDEFS-SF Score Sheet

The subscales of the BDEFS-SF were found to correlate highly with their counterparts on the BDEFS-LF. This was expected, given that only the four highest-loading items from each subscale were used to create the BDEFS-SF. The relationships were as follows: Self-Management to Time (r = .92), Self-Organization/Problem Solving (.92), Self-Restraint (.90), Self-Motivation (.91), and Self-Regulation of Emotion (.94). Thus all patterns of findings concerning the relationship of demographic factors to the BDEFS-LF subscales (see above) were replicated with the BDEFS-SF and its subscales. These results are not reiterated here for space reasons.

The means and standard deviations for each sex within each age group are shown in Table 5.5, along with the results for the two-way (age × sex) analysis of variance that was used to analyze these scores. As can be seen here, significant differences due to age group existed on all scales. Therefore, the scores for the BDEFS-SF

TABLE 5.4. BDEFS-LF Results for Each of the Final Four Age Groups Used to Create the Score Sheets in the Appendix

	Age groups									
	(1) 18–34		(2) 35–49		(3) 50–64		(4) 65–81			
Score/sex	Mean	*SD*	Mean	*SD*	Mean	*SD*	Mean	*SD*	*F*	*p*
Self-Organize	36.7	12.3	34.7	12.6	36.5	12.1	36.1	9.6	G = 1.83	NS
Males	36.6	12.4	34.4	12.8	35.8	12.4	35.7	9.8	S = 1.49	NS
Females	36.8	11.1	35.1	12.3	37.4	12.0	36.4	9.4	G × S = 0.19	NS
Time Mgmt.	36.7	11.8	33.7	11.5	34.4	10.7	32.2	8.1	G = 9.22 1 > 2,3,4 3 > 4	< .001
Males	37.0	12.6	34.0	12.4	34.1	10.5	32.5	8.6	S = 0.23	NS
Females	36.5	10.8	33.4	10.6	34.7	11.0	31.9	7.5	G × S = 0.25	NS
Self-Restraint	30.0	9.6	27.8	9.1	28.6	7.9	27.4	6.6	G = 5.25 1 > 2,3,4	.001
Males	30.7	10.1	28.2	10.0	28.8	8.8	28.0	6.3	S = 4.21 M > F	.040
Females	29.3	9.0	27.5	8.1	28.3	6.9	26.8	6.8	G × S = 0.18	NS
Emotion Reg.	20.5	8.0	19.7	8.0	19.0	6.3	18.2	5.2	G = 5.82 1 > 3,4 2 > 4	.001
Males	19.8	8.2	19.4	8.1	18.5	6.5	18.2	5.3	S = 3.30	NS
Females	21.2	7.8	20.0	7.9	19.5	6.1	18.1	5.1	G × S = 0.68	NS
Self-Motivate	16.5	5.8	15.2	5.2	15.3	4.8	14.4	3.1	G = 9.19 1 > 2,3,4 3 > 4	< .001
Males	17.1	6.1	15.8	6.0	15.9	5.6	14.6	3.2	S = 14.27 M > F	< .001
Females	15.8	5.4	14.5	4.1	14.8	3.9	14.1	3.0	G × S = 0.39	NS
EF Summary	140.4	40.0	131.1	40.3	133.9	36.0	128.3	26.3	G = 6.04 1 > 2,3,4	< .001
Males	141.1	42.6	131.8	43.5	133.2	38.1	129.1	27.9	S = 0.14	NS
Females	139.7	37.4	130.4	37.0	134.6	34.0	127.4	24.6	G × S = 0.13	NS
EF Symptoms	10.2	14.7	7.3	13.5	7.0	12.1	4.5	6.9	G = 10.64	< .001
Males	10.5	15.8	8.4	14.8	7.2	12.7	4.8	7.0	S = 1.70	NS
Females	9.9	13.5	6.3	12.0	6.9	11.5	4.2	6.8	G × S = 0.32 1 > 2,3,4 2 > 4; 3 > 4	NS

Note. See footnote to Table 5.1 for explanations. In addition, EF Symptoms, EF Symptom Count; G, main effect for age group; S, main effect for sex; G × S, interaction of age group × sex. If the main effect for age group was significant, pairwise contrasts are indicated by the number of each age group; for instance, 1 > 2,3,4 means that Group 1 (ages 18–34) had significantly higher scores than did Groups 2, 3, and 4, which did not differ from each other. If the main effect for sex was significant, the contrast of males against females is shown as, for instance, M > F.

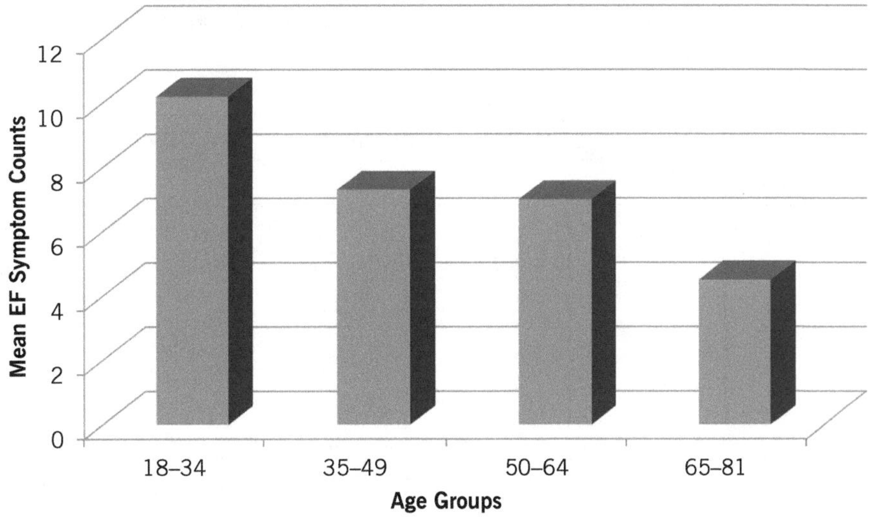

FIGURE 5.9. Mean number of EF symptoms endorsed by each age group. A symptom is counted if the item was answered as occurring often (3) or very often (4).

are shown in the Appendix broken down by age group. Significant sex differences emerged on just two of the subscales, and a third approached significance. However, inspection of the mean differences showed them to be relatively trivial as far as presentation of the BDEFS-SF norms was concerned. Inspection of the distributions for each sex within each age showed this to be the case as well: The cut-off points for the 90th, 95th, and 98th percentiles were almost always identical. Therefore, the score sheet for the BDEFS-SF in the Appendix gives just the breakdown by age. As on the score sheets for the BDEFS-LF, raw score ranges are presented for the 1st–25th, 26th–50th, and 51st–75th percentiles; above the 75th percentile, raw scores for specific percentiles are given. The Total EF Summary Score is considered to be the most valid BDEFS-SF score; that is, it is considered the most representative of the normative population, compared to the scores for the subscales on this form.

TABLE 5.5. BDEFS-SF Results for Each of the Final Four Age Groups Used to Create the Score Sheet in the Appendix

	Age groups									
	(1) 18–34		(2) 35–49		(3) 50–64		(4) 65–81			
Score/sex	Mean	*SD*	Mean	*SD*	Mean	*SD*	Mean	*SD*	*F*	*p*
Self-Organize	5.7	2.2	5.6	2.3	6.0	2.3	6.1	1.9	G = 3.65	.012
Males	5.7	2.4	5.5	2.3	5.8	2.3	6.0	1.9	S = 3.56	NS
Females	5.7	2.0	5.7	2.3	6.3	2.4	6.2	2.0	G × S = 0.65	NS
									1 > 4	
									2 > 3,4	
Time Mgmt.	7.7	2.8	7.1	2.7	7.2	2.5	6.9	2.1	G = 8.04	< .001
Males	7.6	3.0	7.1	2.8	7.3	2.4	6.7	2.2	S = 0.4	NS
Females	7.8	2.7	7.0	2.7	7.1	2.6	6.6	2.0	G × S = 0.26	NS
									1 > 2,3,4	
									3 > 4	
Self-Restraint	6.1	2.3	5.7	2.1	6.0	2.0	5.7	1.7	G = 3.15	.024
Males	6.2	2.4	5.8	2.3	5.9	2.1	5.8	1.7	S = 0.76	NS
Females	6.0	2.2	5.6	1.9	6.1	1.9	5.5	1.7	G × S = 0.68	NS
									1 > 2,4	
Emotion Reg.	6.3	2.9	6.1	2.7	5.7	2.2	5.5	1.9	G = 6.56	< .001
Males	6.0	2.9	6.0	2.8	5.6	2.3	5.4	2.0	S = 3.75	.053
Females	6.6	2.9	6.1	2.7	5.9	2.2	5.5	1.9	G × S = 0.66	NS
									F > M	
									1 > 3,4	
									2 > 4	
Self-Motivate	5.2	1.9	4.8	1.7	4.8	1.7	4.4	0.9	G = 12.91	< .001
Males	5.4	2.0	5.0	2.0	5.0	2.0	4.4	0.9	S = 10.15	.001
Females	5.1	1.8	4.6	1.3	4.6	1.2	4.4	0.9	G × S = 0.59	NS
									M > F	
									1 > 2,3,4	
									2 > 4, 3 > 4	
EF Summary	31.1	9.2	29.2	9.2	29.8	8.4	28.3	6.1	G = 5.67	.001
Males	31.0	9.6	29.4	9.9	29.6	8.8	28.4	6.5	S = 0.00	NS
Females	31.2	8.9	29.0	8.5	30.0	8.0	28.2	5.7	G × S = 0.13	NS
									1 > 2,4	
									3 > 4	
EF Symptoms	2.2	3.3	1.7	3.1	1.6	2.9	0.9	1.8	G = 9.34	< .001
Males	2.2	3.5	1.9	3.4	1.7	3.0	1.0	1.8	S = 0.92	NS
Females	2.3	3.2	1.4	2.8	1.5	2.8	0.9	1.8	G × S = 0.57	NS

Note. See footnotes to Tables 5.1 and 5.4 for explanations.

CHAPTER 6

Reliability

This brief chapter presents the information that is available concerning the various forms of reliability for the BDEFS. Obviously, more research on these and other psychometric characteristics of the scale is to be encouraged. But what information is available indicates that the reliability of the BDEFS is satisfactory for its use in clinical practice and research where the assessment of EF in daily life activities is of interest.

Subscale Relationships

As indicated by the factor analysis reported in Chapter 4, ratings of EF in daily life activities appear to tap a large underlying dimension that mainly consists of self-organization, problem solving, and self-management in relation to time. This dimension is partially coupled to several related yet separable dimensions that deal not only with these constructs, but also with self-restraint (inhibition), self-motivation, and the self-regulation of emotion. We should therefore not be surprised to find that the BDEFS subscales created from all these dimensions are likewise interrelated yet partially separable.

This was evaluated by computing Pearson product–moment correlations among the five BDEFS-LF subscales and the ADHD-EF Index, using the entire normative sample of 1,249 participants. The results are shown in Table 6.1 and indicate that these scores were significantly and moderately intercorrelated. The strongest relationship was between Self-Restraint and Self-Regulation of Emotion (.768). This is understandable, given that the two steps in emotional self-control have been

TABLE 6.1. Intercorrelations among the BDEFS-LF Subscales and ADHD-EF Index

	Self-Organize	Time Mgmt.	Self-Restraint	Emotion Reg.	Self-Motivate	ADHD
Self-Organize	1.00					
Time Mgmt.	.696	1.00				
Self-Restraint	.684	.601	1.00			
Emotion Reg.	.625	.545	.768	1.00		
Self-Motivate	.604	.658	.644	.578	1.00	
ADHD	.764	.875	.797	.673	.775	1.00

Note. Self-Organize, Self-Organization/Problem Solving subscale; Time Mgmt., Self-Management to Time subscale; Emotion Reg., Self-Regulation of Emotion subscale; Self-Motivate, Self-Motivation subscale; ADHD, ADHD-EF Index. All correlations are statistically significant at $p < .001$.

argued to be initial inhibition followed by subsequent efforts at self-management of the emotional state, as discussed in earlier chapters. The weakest relationship occurred between Self-Management to Time and Self-Regulation of Emotion. The shared variance among the subscales ranges from 29.7% to 58.9%; this implies that there is likely to be an underlying unitary construct of EF (perhaps comparable to *g* in research on intelligence tests), yet with some unique variance accounted for by each subscale apart from the others.

These results are comparable to those found in the UMASS Study (Barkley et al., 2008) for the P-BDEFS, where the relationships were of an even higher magnitude, due to the overrepresentation of adults with ADHD and adults with other clinical disorders in which high levels of EF problems would be expected (Barkley & Murphy, 2010b). The intercorrelations ranged from .74 to .88 for the self-ratings and .75 to .88 for the other-ratings. The subscales shared 56–77% of their variance. This was also the case for the interview version of the P-BDEFS when used in our study of ADHD's persistence into adulthood, known as the Milwaukee Study (Barkley & Fischer, in press; Barkley et al., 2008). There the five P-BDEFS dimensions were significantly intercorrelated, with results for each subscale as follows: Self-Management to Time correlated .66 to .77 with the other subscales; Self-Organization/Problem Solving, .63 to .71; Self-Restraint, .67 to .75; Self-Motivation, .63 to .77; and Self-Activation, .66 to .75 (all p's < .001). There was substantial shared variance among the subscales, ranging from 40% to 59%. Thus, as noted in previous chapters, the evidence indicates that EF is both a unitary construct and a diverse one with several interrelated yet semi-independent components.

The ADHD-EF Index from the BDEFS-LF related well to all of these components of EF (see Table 6.1), given that items for this 11-item index were pulled from the BDEFS subscales (except for Self-Regulation of Emotion). The BDEFS-SF was found to correlate highly with the BDEFS-LF ($r = .97$, $p < .001$).

As noted previously, an interview version of the P-BDEFS was created for our prior studies. When factor-analyzed, it yielded the same factor structure as the rating scale (Barkley & Fischer, in press). In Chapter 2, correlations were reported between the factor scores from the P-BDEFS interview and those for the P-BDEFS rating scale, since both were collected on the same samples in the UMASS Study of adult ADHD. The results showed that the scores for each of the factors and for the sum of all factor scores were highly correlated between these two measures: Self-Management to Time (r = .921), Self-Organization/Problem Solving (.885), Self-Restraint (.873), Self-Motivation (.867), Self-Activation/Concentration (.904), and the Total EF Summary Score (.925). All correlations were significant at p < .001. The high magnitude of these relationships makes it likely that any of the findings discussed here concerning the rating scale form would be comparable for the interview form.

Interobserver Agreement and Disparity

Two versions of the BDEFS-LF rating scale and two of the BDEFS-SF are provided in the present manual; one version of each scale is for obtaining self-reports, and the other for collecting the reports of others about the individual being evaluated. Only the Self-Report forms were used to collect the normative information provided in this manual. The Other-Report forms are useful in evaluating the degree of disparity or agreement between the self-reported information and the information provided by a collateral person who knows the patient or research participant well. Information was collected in the UMASS Study on the P-BDEFS from both sources (Barkley & Murphy, 2010b). The correlations between self- and other-ratings were as follows: Self-Management to Time (r = .79, p < .001); Self-Organization/Problem Solving (r = .66, p < .001); Self-Restraint (r = .74, p < .001); and Self-Motivation (r = .69, p < .001). (Recall that the P-BDEFS did not have a subscale assessing self-regulation of emotion.) This suggests a reasonable level of agreement between self- and other-ratings of EF on the four subscales of the P-BDEFS that are the direct ancestors of subscales on the BDEFS.

In the UMASS Study, we also examined the degree of disparity between the P-BDEFS self-ratings and other-ratings by calculating difference scores between the two sets of ratings. The typical disparity averaged just < 1 to 2 points on the subscales of the P-BDEFS for the Community control group (n's = 82–87), which was the group most comparable to the normative sample being reported here. But there were relatively large standard deviations around the means for this group. The mean disparities and standard deviations for each of the four relevant P-BDEFS subscales were as follows: Self-Management to Time (M = 0.7, SD = 8.2); Self-Organization/Problem Solving (M = 2.0, SD = 6.0); Self-Restraint (M = –0.7, SD = 7.1); and Self-Motivation (M = –0.01, SD = 3.0). This suggests that, on average, individuals in a general community sample slightly overestimate their EF ratings relative to those who know them well on the first two of these subscales, while very slightly underestimating their EF problems on the other two. The disparity scores in the two clinical groups (ADHD and Clinical control) were, of course, significantly higher than these mean disparity scores, owing in part to the fact that these clinical groups had high ratings of EF problems. This created an opportunity for a wider disparity between their ratings and those provided by others. The two clinical groups did not differ in their mean disparity scores, and both groups reported more EF problems across these four subscales than did others who knew them well.

Because the individual disparity scores can be either positive (indicating an overestimate in the self-ratings relative to the other-ratings) or negative (indicating an underestimate), these average disparity scores may be canceling out a wider range of absolute disparities. Computation of the absolute disparity scores (regardless of direction) indicated this to be the case. The mean absolute disparity scores were as follows: Self-Management to Time (M = 5.0, SD = 6.5); Self-Organization/Problem Solving (M = 3.9, SD = 5.0); Self-Restraint (M = 4.5, SD = 5.5); and Self-Motivation (M = 1.7, SD = 2.7). These disparities were not correlated with either age or IQ in the data from the UMASS project.

There were moderate and significant correlations with self-rated severity of ADHD, anxiety, and depression, suggesting that individuals reporting higher levels of those internalizing scores were also likely to have greater disparities between their own reports and those of others who knew them well. For ADHD ratings, these correlations were as follows: Self-Management to Time (r = .27, p < .001); Self-Organization/Problem Solving (r = .46, p < .001); Self-Restraint (r = .34, p = .014); and Self-Motivation (r = .40, p < .001). For depression ratings, these correlations were the following: Self-Management to Time (r = .33, p < .001); Self-Organization/Problem Solving (r = .50, p < .001); Self-Restraint (r = .27, p < .001); and Self-Motivation (r = .41, p < .001). And for anxiety, these correlations were as follows: Self-Management to Time (r = .31, p < .001); Self-Organization/Problem Solving (r = .47, p < .001); Self-Restraint (r = .25, p < .001); and Self-Motivation (r = .37, p < .001). These correlations would be expected to be higher than those to be found in a normative sample drawn from the general population, such as that described in this manual for the BDEFS. This is because of the substantial overrepresentation of clinic-referred patients in this earlier study of the P-BDEFS, in which over 65% of the participants had either ADHD or another clinical diagnosis, with the remainder representing the Community control group.

When we examined the correlations with self-rated ADHD, anxiety, and depression for just the Community control group in the UMASS Study, the results were more modest and (for anxiety and depression) often not significant. For ADHD ratings, the correlations were as follows: Self-Management to Time (r = .43, p < .001); Self-Organization/Problem Solving (r = .47, p < .001); Self-Restraint (r = .28, p = .014); and Self-Motivation (r = .39, p < .001). For depression, they were the following: Self-Management to Time (r = .19, p = NS); Self-Organization/Problem Solving (r = .41, p < .001); Self-Restraint (r = .17, p = NS); and Self-Motivation (r = .07, p = NS). And for anxiety, they were as follows: Self-Management to Time (r = .17, p = NS); Self-Organization/Problem Solving (r = .18, p = NS); Self-Restraint (r = .05, p = NS); and Self-Motivation (r = .02, p = NS). These results suggest that in a general community sample, ADHD severity may be related to the degree of disparity seen in self- and other-ratings. But anxiety and depression levels may not be related to most disparities in BDEFS scores, except for a relationship between depression and Self-Organization/Problem Solving. However, among clinic-referred samples in which a psychiatric diagnosis of ADHD or another disorder may exist, the degree of disparities between self- and other-ratings may well be partially a function of the degree of ADHD, anxiety, and depression. This is not to suggest that anxiety and depression may be causing the disparity in self- and other-ratings to increase, only that they are potential correlates of such disparities. It is just as possible that level of EF problems in the patient may be contributing to increased anxiety and depression, either directly or via the adverse effects of EF deficits (and related ADHD symptoms) on adaptive functioning in major life activities (Barkley & Fischer, in press; Barkley & Murphy, 2010a).

In view of the findings described above, clinicians comparing the self-ratings on the BDEFS to ratings provided by others should expect some disparity between these ratings. When would such a disparity be clinically significant? That is, when would it be greater than what would normally be expected? Most likely, this would occur when a disparity between the self- and other-ratings is at least 1 *SD* above these means, which would represent the 84th percentile for disparity scores. This would suggest an unusual level of disagreement, and its likely basis would be worth exploring further clinically in an interview with the client. Given the UMASS Study's findings, the clinician may wish to pay attention to the possibility that ADHD, anxiety, and depression may be comorbid problems when disparity scores exceed this range, particularly if the client is a clinically referred adult. For the BDEFS-LF subscales that have P-BDEFS antecedents, these would be the cutoff points: Self-Management to Time, 11.5 or approximately 12 points; Self-Organization/Problem Solving, 8.9 or approximately 9 points; Self-Restraint, 10 points; and Self-Motivation, 4.4 or approximately 5 points. Disparities on the Self-Regulation of Emotion subscale have not been previously studied, and so no guidance for this subscale can be given. This is also true for the BDEFS-SF. However, given its exceptionally high correlation with the BDEFS-LF, one could argue that all of the findings here that apply to the BDEFS-LF Total EF Summary Score could be expected to apply to the corresponding score for the BDEFS-SF.

Internal Consistency

The internal consistency of each BDEFS-LF subscale (Cronbach's alpha) was found to be satisfactory: Self-Management to Time, .949; Self-Organization/Problem Solving, .958; Self-Restraint, .930; Self-Motivation, .914; and Self-Regulation of Emotion, .946. For the ADHD-EF Index, it was .842, and for the BDEFS-LF Total EF Summary Score, it was .918. All *F*-tests were significant at $p < .001$. Such results are quite comparable to those for other rating scales of EF in adults (e.g., the BRIEF; Roth et al., 2005). Since norms are not available for the Other-Report forms of the present BDEFS, information on the internal consistency of their subscales cannot be examined. But such reports are available for the P-BDEFS in the UMASS Study (Barkley et al., 2008).

Test–Retest Reliability

Test–retest reliability was assessed by having a subset of 62 adults complete the BDEFS-LF on a second occasion 2–3 weeks after initially completing the scale. Half of the 10 participants at each age level were men, and half were women. These adults were randomly chosen by Knowledge Networks within each age group and sex, and were invited to return to the website to complete the scale for a second time. They were, of course, paid for their participation, just as were all participants on the first occasion of assessment.

The Pearson product–moment correlations between the first and second administrations were as follows: Self-Management to Time, .83 (p < .001); Self-Organization/Problem Solving, .90 (p < .001); Self-Restraint, .78 (p < .001); Self-Motivation, .62 (p < .001); Self-Regulation of Emotion, .78 (p < .001); and the Total EF Summary Score, .84 (p < .001). The test–retest reliability for the ADHD-EF Index was .76 (p < .001), and that for the BDEFS-SF Total EF Summary Score was .80 (p < .001). These results are quite satisfactory and indicate a reasonable level of test–retest reliability over this 2- to 3-week period. They are also relatively comparable to the test–retest reliability found for another rating scale of EF for adults (the BRIEF) over an average 4-week interval (Roth et al., 2005).

The actual scores from the initial testing and retesting administrations were then compared via a paired-samples t-test. The results are shown in Table 6.2. They indicate that the BDEFS-LF subscale scores, Total EF Summary Score, ADHD-EF Index, and the BDEFS-SF Total EF Summary Score, did not change significantly across this 2- to 3-week test–retest interval. Again, this supports the conclusion that both the BDEFS-LF and BDEFS-SF have satisfactory test–retest reliability, with no evidence of significant changes in results over this interval of time.

TABLE 6.2. Comparison of Initial and Retesting Sample Results on BDEFS Scores (n = 62)

	Initial		Retesting				
Score	Mean	*SD*	Mean	*SD*	Mean diff.	*t*	*p*
Time Mgmt.	34.0	10.9	32.7	11.5	1.35	1.61	NS
Self-Organize	35.4	12.3	35.2	12.8	0.24	0.34	NS
Self-Restraint	28.7	9.7	28.3	9.3	0.42	0.52	NS
Self-Motivate	15.7	4.9	15.3	4.6	0.42	0.79	NS
Emotion Reg.	20.0	7.0	19.2	7.3	0.76	1.25	NS
BDEFS-LF EF Summary	133.9	38.6	130.7	40.4	3.19	1.11	NS
ADHD	16.8	5.4	16.2	5.1	0.53	1.16	NS
BDEFS-SF EF Summary	29.9	9.2	29.0	9.1	0.98	1.36	NS

Note. See footnote to Table 6.1 for explanations. In addition, EF Summary, Total EF Summary Score; Mean diff., differences in the initial and retesting means; t, results for the paired-samples t-test; p, probability value for the t-test if ≤ .05; NS, not significant.

CHAPTER 7

Validity

"Validity" refers to the correctness, accuracy, or truth of an assertion or conclusion, typically as measured against the empirical evidence in support of or refuting the assertion (Bryant, 2000). In the case of measurement, "validity" refers to the extent to which the measure does what it claims to do. In the present case, it refers to the extent to which the BDEFS is measuring EF in daily life activities and to its usefulness (utility) in doing so. Much of the work of validating the BDEFS was done over the previous decade with the P-BDEFS. The content of the two scales is highly similar, in that the vast majority of items on each of the P-BDEFS subscales also appeared in the final BDEFS (see Chapter 4). Only the Self-Regulation of Emotion subscale of the BDEFS had no equivalent on the P-BDEFS, and so its validity is not as well established. However, as will be shown below, what evidence exists for this newer subscale shows that it is as valid as the other subscales.

Construct Validity

Establishing construct validity must begin with explicitly and clearly defining the construct that a measure is intended to assess (Bryant, 2000; Cook & Campbell, 1979). Otherwise, one cannot determine whether the measure is accurately or correctly sampling from and hence evaluating the conceptual domain of this construct. Despite the widespread use of the term "EF," it has not been especially well defined, as noted in Chapter 1. Therefore, any effort to evaluate the construct validity of any measure of EF has been hampered by the ambiguity in and lack of any consensus in defining the term.

Relationship to EF Tests

Let us consider the use of putative EF tests, such as continuous performance tests (CPTs), digit span backward tests, or even the venerable Wisconsin Card Sorting Test (WCST). From their content, one would think that EF is defined as attention, inhibition, short-term memory and manipulation, or rule discovery, respectively. Yet the most often cited definition of EF, particularly in recent research in ADHD, is typically something to this effect: those neurocognitive processes necessary for sustaining goal-directed problem solving. One can rightly ask, "Just where is goal-directed problem solving sampled in these various EF tests?" And just what makes a measure of inhibition or short-term memory a neurocognitive process essential to such goal-directed problem solving? The point here is not to revisit the issues raised in earlier chapters concerning the serious problems with past and present definitions of the term "EF." But it is to illustrate that evaluating the construct validity of any newly proposed measure of EF, such as the BDEFS, is going to be hampered if the prior vague and diverse definitions of EF are to be used to evaluate such validity.

As a consequence of their numerous inherent problems (see Chapter 2), EF tests cannot be used as the gold standard against which to evaluate a new measure of EF—in this case, a rating scale of EF in everyday activities. It is questionable whether the wide array of tests claimed to be evaluating EF in neuropsychology can meet acceptable standards themselves for construct validity, much less serve as the standard against which any new measure of EF is to be judged. As previously noted, tests of EF are poorly correlated with rating scales of EF in daily life activities and are equally poor at predicting functioning and impairment in major life activities in which EF would be considered indispensable. EF tests, therefore, should not be used as the standard for evaluating the construct validity of any new measure of EF, especially a rating scale, given the substantial evidence already available as to their own low construct and especially ecological validity. The prevailing evidence suggests that the problem here rests with the tests more than with the rating scales of EF, especially if predicting functioning and impairment in major life activities is the clinical objective in the evaluation of EF.

As noted previously, our research with the P-BDEFS did examine its relationship to several different brief batteries of EF tests (Barkley & Fischer, in press; Barkley & Murphy, 2010b). These tests are described in Box 7.1 and included tests of inhibition and attention (the Conners CPT); the Stroop Color–Word Test to examine interference control (distractibility); digit span, paragraph comprehension, and word-pair-learning tasks to assess verbal working memory; spatial and sequential memory tasks to evaluate nonverbal working memory; the WCST to evaluate problem solving and rule discovery; the Tower of London Test (TOL) to assess planning and problem solving; and verbal and nonverbal fluency tests, such as the Five-Points Test. The correlations between the P-BDEFS subscales and these tests are shown in Table 7.1 for the large UMASS Study of adults with ADHD, and in Table 7.2 for the Milwaukee Study of hyperactive children followed to adulthood.

(text resumes on page 77)

BOX 7.1. Neuropsychological Tests of EF Utilized in the UMASS and Milwaukee Studies

Various neuropsychological tests of EF were used to evaluate their associations with the P-BDEFS in my prior research with my colleagues discussed in this chapter. That research is described in detail in Barkley and colleagues (2008). Here those tests are described for readers unfamiliar with them.

EF TESTS USED IN THE UMASS STUDY OF ADULTS WITH ADHD

- *Conners Continuous Performance Test (Conners, 1995).* This is a standardized computer-administered CPT in which single letters are shown on a display screen at three different rates: one every second, one every 2 seconds, or one every 4 seconds. The task lasts 12 minutes. The variation in interstimulus interval allows the effects of this variable on the participant's performance to be examined. The task uses a response format that is the reverse of most CPTs: The participant presses a button in response to every signal shown, but then must cease or inhibit their responding when the target signal appears. The dependent measures employed here were the total number of Omissions (missed targets), total Commissions (false hits), Reaction Time (RT), and RT Variability. The scores for Omissions and RT Variability were chosen to assess sustained attention, while the scores for Commissions and RT were chosen to assess response inhibition. We previously reported the group differences on this test (Barkley et al., 2008): We found the group with ADHD to score significantly worse than the Community control group on all measures, and worse than the Clinical control group on Omissions and RT Variability.
- *Stroop Color–Word Test (Stroop, 1935; Trenerry, Crosson, Deboe, & Leber, 1989).* This test measures the ability to inhibit competing responses in the presence of salient conflicting information. The version and norms published by Trenerry and colleagues (1989) were used here. The task has three parts. In the first part, the participant reads a repeating list of color names (e.g., red, blue, green) printed in black ink. In the second part, the participant names the colors of a repeated series of ×'s printed in inks of those same colors. In the last or Interference condition, the participant must say the color of the ink in which a color word is printed. For some words, the color of the ink in which it is printed is the same as that of the word; for others, the color of ink differs from that specified by the word. This portion of the task is believed to reflect problems with the capacity to inhibit habitual or dominant responses (reading the word, in this case). Three scores were derived from this last portion of the test (Interference): the raw scores for the number of items completed and the number of incorrect responses, as well as the percentile score. We previously reported the group comparisons on this test (Barkley et al., 2008): We found just the ADHD group to differ from the Community control group. Only the percentile score was used here.
- *Wisconsin Card Sorting Test (WCST; Heaton, 1981).* This test comprises 128 cards, each containing sets of geometric designs that vary according to color, shape, and number. The subject is given four cards and is then asked to sort the remaining deck, using feedback from the examiner. Following 10 correct sorts on a given category (e.g., color), the examiner switches the category unannounced, and the subject must now discover the new sorting rule from feedback given by the examiner. Although many scores can be derived, we used just five: the scores for percent Errors, percent Perseverative Errors, Concepts, Categories Achieved, and Failures to Maintain Set. We previously reported the comparisons among these groups on this test; none were significant (Barkley et al., 2008).

(cont.)

• *Five-Points Test of Design Fluency (Lee et al., 1997).* Originally developed by Regard, Strauss, and Knapp (1982) as an attempt to design a nonverbal version of more commonly used verbal working memory and fluency tasks, this test involves a sheet of paper with 40 five-dot matrices on it. Participants are required to produce as many different figures as possible by connecting the dots within each rectangle within a 3-minute time limit. Not all dots have to be used, and only straight lines between dots are permitted. No figures are to be repeated. If a violation occurs, participants are given a single warning on the first violation, but the rules are not repeated after any further infractions. Scores are the number of unique designs created, the number of repeated designs (perseveration), the number of rule infractions, and the percentage of designs that are repeated designs (percent perseveration). Patients with frontal lobe dysfunction have a significantly higher percentage of perseverative errors than do either neurological patients without frontal involvement or psychiatric patients (Lee et al., 1997). Using a modified version of this same task, Ruff, Allen, Farrow, Nieman, and Wylie (1994) also found the task to be sensitive to frontal lobe injuries, and perhaps more sensitive to right- than to left-lobe involvement. Here we used just the Unique Designs measure (number of unique designs generated in the task). We have previously reported significant group differences on this test score among these three groups (Barkley et al., 2008).

• *Learning and Memory Battery (LAMB; Multi-Health Systems, 1995).* This battery contains nine separate tests involving verbal learning, verbal memory, and nonverbal memory. Multiple test scores are derived from these various tests (at least three per test), but most reflect learning and memory retention. We found significant group differences for most of the memory retention scores from this battery, and have reported the group differences for the entire LAMB elsewhere (Barkley et al., 2008). Here we used just the Digit Span (total forward and backward score) as our index of verbal working memory. Each digit string is presented twice, with recall attempted after each presentation. In the first task, respondents must recall the digit sequence as presented. In the second task, they must recall the digit sequences read to them in backward order. In our earlier comparisons of the UMASS groups on this specific subtest, we found the group with ADHD to perform worse than both the Clinical and Community control groups, which did not differ from each other.

EF TESTS USED IN THE MILWAUKEE STUDY OF HYPERACTIVE CHILDREN FOLLOWED TO ADULTHOOD

• *Stroop Color–Word Test (Trenerry et al., 1989).* See description above.

• *Digit Span test from the Wechsler Adult Intelligence Scale—Third Edition (WAIS-III; Wechsler, 1997).* This test served as our measure of verbal working memory. It involves two subtests. In one, the examinee is given a series of increasingly longer strings of digits by the examiner at a rate of one per second. The examiner must repeat them back in the same numerical sequence. In the second subtest, the examinee must repeat increasingly longer strings of digits in the reverse order from that given by the examiner. For both tests, the participant is given two trials at each span length. The test ends when the participant fails to repeat both trials correctly at that span length. The score is the longest span length performed correctly on at least one of the two trials. The raw scores from both tests were combined to form a single raw score, used here.

(cont.)

• *Kaufman Hand Movements (KHM) test from the Kaufman Brief Intelligence Test (Kaufman & Kaufman, 1993).* We employed the KHM as a measure of nonverbal working memory. It is a well-standardized test for children based on a traditional measure of frontal lobe function in adults. Children are presented with progressively longer sequences of three hand movements, which they must imitate. We used the scores for number correct and longest sequence completed.

• *Simon Game.* This task was chosen so as to evaluate nonverbal working memory in a manner equivalent to a digit span forward task. We have used it previously for this purpose with adults who had ADHD, with some success in differentiating that group from control groups (Murphy, Barkley, & Bush, 2001). The task is a commercially available game that consists of a circular plastic device housing four large colored keys on its top surface. When depressed, each of these keys emits a different tone. When activated, the game automatically presents a sequence of different tones and lights up the key corresponding to each tone as it does so. A participant must then press the keys in their correct sequence so as to reproduce the melody. With each trial, the sequence of tone–key combinations becomes increasingly longer and thus more complex. The score used here was the longest correctly reproduced sequence. It is akin to self-ordered pointing tasks (see Lezak et al., 2004). Participants were given two trials at each level of the game (Levels I–IV).

• *Five-Points Test of Design Fluency (Lee et al., 1997).* See description above.

• *Tower of London Test (TOL; Shallice & Burgess, 1991).* This test served as our measure of planning and problem solving. It presents the participant with a stand that contains three upright spindles of different heights, along with three balls of different colors (red, blue, green) that are arranged on two of these spindles. The participant is then shown a diagram illustrating the goal or final position in which these balls are to be rearranged. In proceeding to rearrange the balls in that position, the participant must do so in the fewest moves. The TOL requires that participants look ahead to determine the proper order of moves, and so it is considered a test of planning ability. The test has been used in several neuropsychological studies of children and adults with ADHD, where deficits have been noted (Frazier et al., 2004; Hervey et al., 2004).

Both of these studies were biased by oversampling of adults with ADHD and other clinical disorders. These adults might be expected to have more deviant EF scores than a general population sample would. This would result in finding larger-than-usual correlations between EF ratings and EF tests, given the much wider range of scores on both forms of measurement. The results did show that the P-BDEFS subscales were related to some EF tests; however, they indicated that the P-BDEFS was only weakly related, if at all, to any individual test. The P-BDEFS subscales shared less than 10% of their variance with such tests at best, and less than 20% with any best combination of EF tests (see Barkley & Fischer, in press, and Barkley & Murphy, 2010b, for analyses). This cannot be blamed on the relatively small test batteries or on the particular choice of EF tests. Our results are very consistent with a number of other previous studies that used other EF tests and found much the same results (see Chapter 2).

Another way to illustrate this minimal overlap of EF tests and EF ratings is by showing the percentage of patients in each group who placed in the clinically deficient range on each set of measures. The clinically deficient range here was the 93rd percentile (1.5 *SD*s from the control group mean). This was done for both the Milwaukee Study (Barkley & Fischer, in press), the results of which were used to

TABLE 7.1. Correlations between P-BDEFS Subscales (Self-Ratings) and Neuropsychological Tests of EF in the UMASS Study

	P-BDEFS subscales				
EF tests	S-MT	S-OPS	S-RES	S-MOT	S-ACT
CPT Omissions	.157**	.172**	.185**	.199**	.177**
CPT Commissions	.354**	.304**	.331**	.405**	.331**
CPT RT	–.129*	–.102	–.091	–.192**	–.136*
CPT RT Variability	.221*	.219**	.264**	.273**	.210**
WCST Errors	–.009	–.048	–.057	–.020	–.050
WCST Perseverative Errors	–.018	–.033	–.081	–.009	–.050
WCST Concepts	.038	.050	.067	.066	.040
WCST Categories Achieved	–.012	–.038	–.008	–.021	–.036
WCST Failures to Maintain Set	.087	.110	.108	.127*	.076
Stroop Color–Word Interference % score	–.094	–.183	–.106	–.083	–.105
LAMB Digit Span total score	–.111	–.193**	–.092	–.134*	–.151**
LAMB Paragraph Retention	–.122*	–.199**	–.143*	–.166**	–.176**
LAMB Word Pair Learning Delayed Recall	–.109	–.109	–.154**	–.224**	–.161**
Five-Points Test—Unique Designs	–.192**	–.272**	–.228**	–.181**	–.258**

Note. S-MT, Self-Management to Time subscale; S-OPS, Self-Organization/Problem Solving subscale; S-RES, Self-Restraint subscale; S-MOT, Self-Motivation subscale; S-ACT, Self-Activation/Concentration subscale; CPT, Conners Continuous Performance Test; WCST, Wisconsin Card Sorting Test; %, percentile; LAMB, Learning and Memory Battery. Data from Barkley, Murphy, and Fischer (2008).
$^*p < .05$. $^{**}p < .01$.

TABLE 7.2. Correlations between P-BDEFS Subscales and Neuropsychological Tests of EF in the Milwaukee Study

	P-BDEFS subscales				
EF tests	S-MT	S-OPS	S-RES	S-MOT	S-ACT
WAIS-III Digit Span total score	–.171*	–.309**	–.209**	–.145*	–.264*
Simon longest sequence correct	–.110	–.194**	–.226**	–.210**	–.252**
Five-Points Test—Unique Designs	–.032	–.184**	–.174*	–.126	–.151*
Stroop Word–Color Test Interference score	–.109	–.119	–.164*	–.100	–.169*
TOL total score	–.131	–.187**	–.108	–.079	–.065
TOL number correct—first trial	–.141*	–.180*	–.109	–.118	–.112
TOL time to first move	–.056	–.059	–.074	–.052	–.111
KHM number correct	–.121	–.287**	–.238**	–.189**	–.220**
KHM longest sequence	–.117	–.270**	–.218**	–.187**	–.176*

Note. See footnote to Table 7.1 for P-BDEFS subscale abbreviations. In addition, WAIS-III, Wechsler Adult Intelligence Test—Third Edition; Simon, Simon Game; TOL, Tower of London Test; KHM, Kaufman Hand Movements subtest. $n = 203$. Data from Barkley, Murphy, and Fischer (2008).
$^*p < .05$. $^{**}p < .01$.

create the graph appearing in Figure 7.1, and the UMASS Study (Barkley & Murphy, 2010b), the results of which served as the basis for the graph in Figure 7.2. The vast majority of clinic-referred adults with ADHD and of children whose ADHD persisted into adulthood were impaired on the P-BDEFS subscales (left side of each diagram). Yet only a minority of these individuals were impaired on the EF tests (right side of each diagram).

Given the totality of evidence to date, it can be concluded that EF tests have little or no ecological validity as judged against various EF rating scales and observations and ratings of daily adaptive functioning. They also are far less predictive of impairment in various domains of major life activities (e.g., occupational and educational functioning, driving, marriage, and financial management) than are rating scales such as the BDEFS (Barkley & Fischer, in press; Barkley & Murphy, 2010a).

Face Validity

In contrast to this predicament concerning EF tests, the development of the BDEFS is not based on its being representative of any test of EF or even needing to have such a relationship. The BDEFS is based on a specific operational definition of EF as *self-regulation across time for the attainment of future goals, typically in social contexts.*

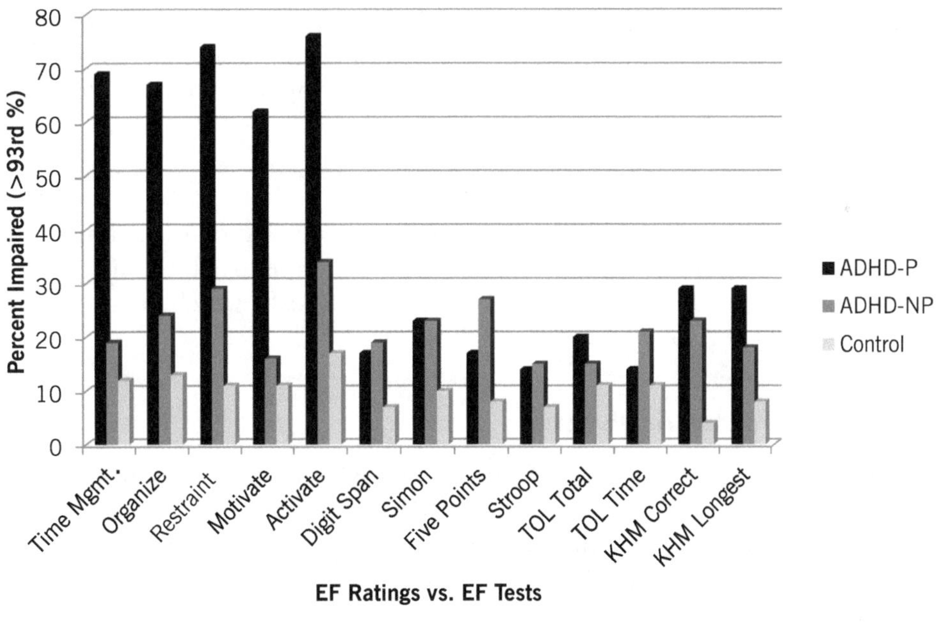

FIGURE 7.1. Percentages of children whose ADHD persisted to age 27 years (ADHD-P), those whose ADHD did not persist (ADHD-NP), and the control group who placed in the clinically impaired range on the five P-BDEFS subscales and the EF test battery in the longitudinal Milwaukee Study. Time Mgmt., Self-Management to Time subscale; Organize, Self-Organization/Problem Solving subscale; Restraint, Self-Restraint subscale; Motivate, Self-Motivation subscale; Activate, Self-Activation/Concentration subscale. See Box 7.1 for explanations of the EF tests. Data from Barkley and Fischer (in press).

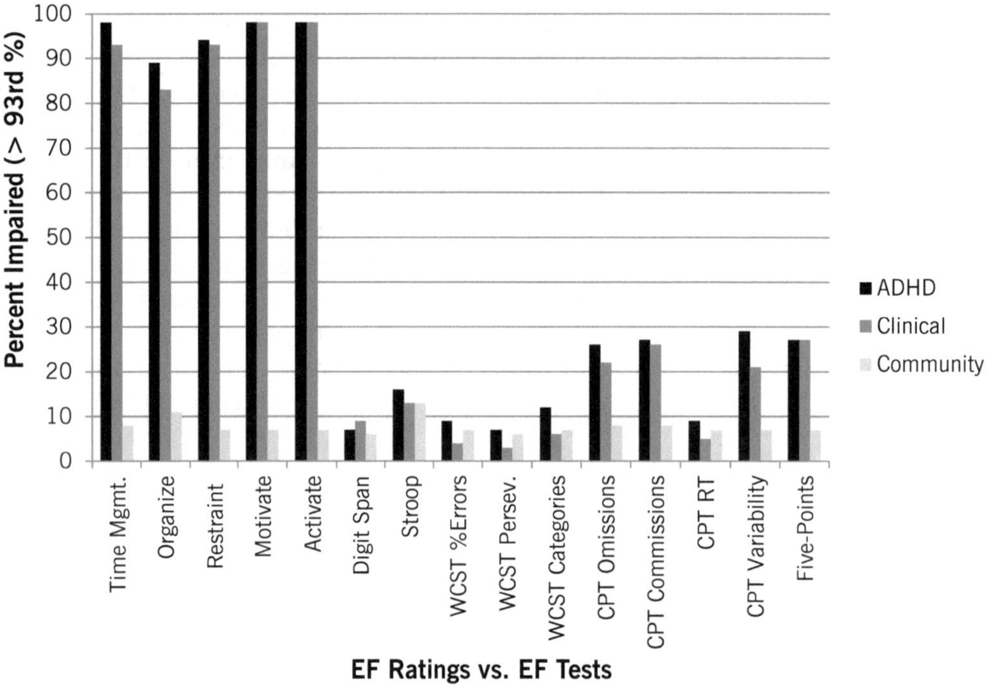

FIGURE 7.2. Percentage of adults with ADHD, Clinical control adults, and Community control adults who placed in the clinically impaired range of the five P-BDEFS subscales and the EF test battery in the UMASS Study. See Figure 7.1 caption and Box 7.1 for explanation. Data from Barkley and Murphy (in press).

The BDEFS was designed to directly assess just such a definition of EF and the neuropsychological components needed to accomplish such self-regulation across time. It therefore has higher face validity than putative EF tests, which, as noted above, are not necessarily developed from the definition of EF.

Evidence from Factor Analyses

Some evidence for how well the BDEFS captures EF became evident in the research conducted over the past decade with the P-BDEFS (Barkley et al., 2008; Barkley & Fischer, in press; Barkley & Murphy, 2010a, 2010b). A factor analysis of the P-BDEFS using the mixed sample of ADHD, Clinical control, and Community control groups in the UMASS Study identified factors labeled as Self-Management to Time, Self-Organization/Problem Solving, Self-Restraint (Inhibition), Self-Motivation, and Self-Activation/Concentration. This same factor structure emerged from the ratings of others on the P-BDEFS concerning the adult participants in that study (Barkley & Murphy, 2010b). And it emerged again in the longitudinal Milwaukee Study of hyperactive children and the persistence of their ADHD into young adulthood (Barkley & Fischer, in press), which employed an interview version of the P-BDEFS. The present research, employing a substantial sample of adults representative of the

U.S. population, found four of these five same factors—with the exception of the Self-Activation/Concentration factor, which was considerably weaker here and consisted of just a few items. Hence it was omitted from further consideration. It probably emerged in the earlier studies related to ADHD because such problems with self-activation may be particularly problematic for that clinical disorder, while not being so evident in a general population sample. It therefore appears that the factor structure of the BDEFS with regard to dimensions representing Self-Management to Time, Self-Organization/Problem Solving, Self-Restraint, and Self-Motivation are reliable features of EF in daily life.

No factor related to emotional self-regulation had the opportunity to emerge in the past research using the P-BDEFS, as items assessing that aspect of EF were not in that prototype. This situation was corrected in the current version of the BDEFS. The correction proved fruitful, as the subsequent factor analysis of the present normative sample revealed just such a dimension of EF in daily life activities, made up of 13 items reflecting problems with emotional inhibition and self-regulation.

All of these efforts at identifying the dimensions underlying the initial large item pool of EF symptoms in daily life suggest that the BDEFS has reasonable construct validity, as judged against the definition of EF offered in Chapter 1. The BDEFS does appear to be assessing self-regulation across time to attain future goals, at least as this may be reflected in survey items focusing on specific forms of behavior. And the scale further evaluates self-organization and problem solving, self-inhibition, self-motivation, and self-regulation of emotion—all of which, as hypothesized, were found to be related (interactive) to varying degrees with this aspect of management of self over time in the role EF plays in daily life activities.

It would surely be informative to determine how well the BDEFS relates to other rating scales of EF, such as the BRIEF or the DEX. No such information was available at this writing (fall 2010). It is left to future researchers to explore that issue. But given the marked similarity of the content of the items among these three scales, at least moderate or stronger relationships are likely to be found. Moreover, the degree of such relationships does not necessarily indicate the construct validity of the BDEFS specifically. The BDEFS is a theoretically—not just an empirically—based rating scale of EF, developed from a particular conceptualization of EF. Because the other EF rating scales were not developed in this way, this will reduce to some degree the magnitude of the relationships to be found between the BDEFS and the other scales.

It will also prove informative for research to evaluate the extent to which various groups with psychiatric and neurological disorders perform on the BDEFS. Some research on adults with ADHD has been done and is described shortly. But it is not essential for the BDEFS to be shown to discriminate patients with frontal lobe disorders as a sine qua non for its construct validity, unless one wishes to regress to an earlier era of research on EF, when it was chiefly believed to represent "what the frontal lobes do." As Denckla (1996) has previously noted, conflating EF (a neuropsychological construct) with any neurological substrate confuses levels of analysis in science and does not provide a solid conceptual basis for further developing and evaluating the concept of EF at the neuropsychological level.

Relationship to IQ and Academic Achievement Skills

Yet another line of evidence supporting the construct validity of the BDEFS comes from prior evidence that it is not significantly associated with IQ or with academic achievement skills to any appreciable degree. This, as noted previously, has posed a considerable problem for EF tests: They are often contaminated by their overlap with general intelligence or with other cognitive constructs not believed to represent EF, such as motor or naming speed. Our earlier work with the P-BDEFS in the UMASS Study found that just one of the five subscales was modestly but significantly correlated with participant IQ, that being Self-Organization/Problem Solving ($r = -.15$, $p = .007$) (Barkley & Murphy, 2010b). The ADHD-EF Index developed in that research was also not significantly correlated with IQ ($r = -.042$, $p =$ NS). This pattern was also the case for the other-ratings on the P-BDEFS ($r = -.17$, $p = .008$). Most P-BDEFS scores were uncorrelated with academic achievement skills as measured by the Wide Range Achievement Test 3 (Jastak & Wilkinson, 1993). Reading was significantly associated with Self-Organization/Problem Solving ($r = -.158$, $p = .005$), as was arithmetic ($r = -.130$, $p = .020$). Spelling was associated only with the Self-Activation/Concentration subscale ($r = -.117$, $p = .034$) (n's = 299–329). The ADHD-EF Index was not significantly correlated with any of these three achievement tests. Yet even when the relationships were significant here, they were weak and indicated that the P-BDEFS subscales shared less than 3% of their variance with certain achievement skills. Thus the P-BDEFS subscales (and, by extension, those of the BDEFS) are largely uncontaminated by general intelligence and academic achievement skills.

Discriminant Validity

As noted above, evidence for the validity of a measure can come from studies of its capacity to distinguish disordered from nondisordered groups, particularly when those disordered groups are believed to have problems with EF. For instance, ADHD is associated with numerous difficulties in EF that are typically assessed with EF tests (Frazier et al., 2004; Hervey et al., 2004; Willcutt et al., 2005). Our research with the P-BDEFS in both the UMASS and Milwaukee Studies found that adults with ADHD had significantly higher ratings on all subscales than did community samples of adults (Barkley & Fischer, in press; Barkley & Murphy, 2010b). They also had higher scores on the P-BDEFS (both the self-report and other-report forms) than did clinic-referred adults (Barkley & Murphy, 2010b). And higher scores on the P-BDEFS were associated with the degree of persistence of ADHD into adulthood in hyperactive children followed longitudinally in the Milwaukee Study, particularly relative to a Community control group (Barkley & Fischer, in press).

As noted above, both of these earlier studies (Barkley & Fischer, in press; Barkley & Murphy, 2010b) also computed the percentages of the various groups that placed in the clinically significant range on the P-BDEFS (above the 93rd percentile). Those results were shown in Figures 7.1 and 7.2. In the UMASS Study of adult ADHD (Barkley & Murphy, in press), results for the self-reports showed that

89–98% of the adults with ADHD placed in this range on the various P-BDEFS subscales, compared to 8–11% of the Community control group. The results for the other-reports placed 84–99% of the ADHD group in this clinically significant range, compared to 7–14% of the Community control group. The study also found that 83–98% of the Clinical control group fell into this range across the various P-BDEFS subscales for the self-reports and 68–89% for the other-ratings. As that study noted, these Clinical control adults had referred themselves to the same adult ADHD clinic believing that they had ADHD, and 45% of them met criteria for that disorder based on their self-reports. But they were judged by an expert clinician not to meet the full DSM-IV criteria for the disorder. Therefore, many in this control group may have had residual ADHD or ADHD not otherwise specified, which would have resulted in their also having high ratings on the P-BDEFS. In addition, they had anxiety disorders, mood disorders, and other psychiatric problems that could be expected to adversely affect EF in daily life activities. And so their elevated rates of placement in the clinically significant range on the P-BDEFS scales were not surprising.

Now let us contrast these results against those obtained with the EF tests. The UMASS Study found that only 7–29% of the ADHD group and 3–27% of the Clinical control group placed above the 93rd percentile compared to the Community control group, whose range of impairment was 6–13%. This evidence indicates that the BDEFS is likely to be useful in discriminating groups of patients with clinical disorders from the general population of adults, and especially useful in identifying adults with ADHD. In contrast, the EF tests were of little value in identifying EF deficits in these clinical populations. Similar patterns of results were evident in the Milwaukee Study of hyperactive children followed into young adulthood (Barkley & Fischer, in press) and in previous studies of patients with frontal lobe injuries (Alderman et al., 2003; Burgess et al., 1998), as discussed earlier.

As for the ADHD-EF Index, results from the UMASS Study (Barkley & Murphy, 2010b) indicated that 98.5% of the group with ADHD surpassed the impairment cutoff of the 93rd percentile, as did 96.6% of the Clinical control group, but just 7.6% of the Community control group. Thus the vast majority of adults with clinically diagnosed ADHD scored in the impaired range on the ADHD-EF Index, much as they did on the larger P-BDEFS from which this index is drawn.

Certainly much work remains to be done on the validity of the BDEFS as a measure of EF in daily life activities. Additional studies using the BDEFS with other groups of patients presumed to have deficits in EF, such as those with obvious neurological disorders previously known to compromise EF, would be informative concerning the scale's discriminant validity. The evidence described above on adults with ADHD, a far more subtle disorder of prefrontal lobe functioning and EF, suggests that such research would prove fruitful. And so does the evidence that is accumulating for the discriminant validity of other rating scales of EF, such as the BRIEF and the DEX, as discussed in Chapter 2. Again, given the content overlap across these rating scales, available evidence would suggest that the BDEFS would prove just as likely to discriminate various clinical groups believed to have impaired EF.

Criterion Validity

Criterion validity is one means of evaluating a measure for its usefulness in assessing a construct. If the measure assesses that construct, then it should be related to future (predictive validity), present (concurrent validity), and past (retrospective validity) outcomes known to be associated with that construct (Bryant, 2000). No information is currently available on the value of the BDEFS in predicting *future* outcomes believed to be associated with EF, such as occupational, educational, financial, social, health, or even criminal outcomes. To determine this value, we would need a longitudinal study following participants for a period of time after the BDEFS was administered and evaluating various outcomes. We could then examine how well baseline scores on the BDEFS predicted these later outcomes. However, there is evidence available on the concurrent validity of the BDEFS (i.e., how closely it was associated with measures of EF-related outcomes collected concurrently with the BDEFS). And there is evidence on its retrospective or postdictive validity (i.e., how closely it was associated with prior outcomes on which information was collected before the BDEFS administration).

Severity of ADHD

In the UMASS and Milwaukee Studies, the extent to which the P-BDEFS was associated with severity of ADHD was examined (Barkley & Fischer, in press; Barkley & Murphy, 2010b). As noted above, ADHD is believed to be associated with significant problems with EF, both in current theorizing about the disorder (Barkley, 1997b, 2006; Castellanos et al., 2006; Nigg & Casey, 2005) and in meta-analyses of research using EF tests (Frazier et al., 2004; Hervey et al., 2004; Nigg, Willcutt, Doyle, & Sonuga-Barke, 2005; Willcutt et al., 2005). In the UMASS Study, as noted above, we found that the vast majority of adults with ADHD placed in the impaired range on the P-BDEFS subscales and the ADHD-EF Index. The ADHD, Clinical, and Community control groups from that study (Barkley & Murphy, 2010b) were combined and examined here for the relationship of P-BDEFS subscales to ADHD severity ratings. The correlations with Inattentive symptoms were as follows: Self-Management to Time (r = .91), Self-Organization/Problem Solving (.80), Self-Restraint (.85), Self-Motivation (.83), and Self-Activation/Concentration (.87). For the ADHD-EF Index, this correlation was just as high (.92). The correlations with Hyperactive–Impulsive symptoms were as follows: Self-Management to Time (r = .71), Self-Organization/Problem Solving (.68), Self-Restraint (.84), Self-Motivation (.71), Self-Activation/Concentration (.80), and ADHD-EF Index (.80). All p's were $< .001$. Such findings indicate near-colinearity of EF problems with ADHD symptoms; in other words, ratings of one construct (EF) are highly related to ratings of the other (ADHD). Indeed, they may well be identifying the same construct.

We conducted a factor analysis using the two ADHD symptom dimensions from the UMASS Study, along with the five P-BDEFS subscales; a promax rotation was employed. The analysis revealed just a single factor having an eigenvalue greater than 1. The factor loadings were these: ADHD Inattentive = .739, ADHD Hyperactive–Impulsive = .630, Self-Management to Time = .912, Self-Organization/Problem Solving = .851, Self-Restraint = .903, Self-Motivation = .897, and Self-Activation/

Concentration = .924. The loadings make it clear that this is an EF dimension, as the highest loadings are from the P-BDEFS. But they also make it clear that EF and ADHD are two views or names for the same common single construct. This obviously supports the view that ADHD is a disorder of EF, especially as manifested in daily life activities such as those evaluated on the P-BDEFS.

We also found in the UMASS Study strong relationships between current P-BDEFS ratings and retrospective self-ratings of ADHD during childhood (ages 5–12 years): Self-Management to Time (r = .72), Self-Organization/Problem Solving (.70), Self-Restraint (.80), Self-Motivation (.72), and Self-Activation/Concentration (.81) (Barkley & Murphy, in press). For the ADHD-EF Index, this relationship was .79. Again, all p's were < .001.

As part of the data collection on the normative sample for the BDEFS, participants also completed an adult ADHD rating scale (Barkley & Murphy, 2006) that contains the 18 items from the DSM-IV criteria for ADHD. Each of the symptoms is rated on a Likert scale from 1 (not at all or rarely) to 4 (very often), which is identical to the item response format for the BDEFS. The symptom scores for this rating scale were summed to create Inattentive, Hyperactive–Impulsive, and Total ADHD Symptom scores. Correlations were then computed between BDEFS scores and each of these ADHD symptom dimensions. The results are shown in Table 7.3. The BDEFS scores correlated more highly, on average, with the Inattentive dimension than with the Hyperactive–Impulsive dimension of ADHD symptoms except for the Self-Restraint and Self-Regulation of Emotion subscales, both of which have items that are more similar to the construct of impulsiveness than to that of inattention. All correlations were based on the entire sample of 1,249 adults, and all p's were < .001.

To reinforce the point that ADHD symptoms and EF deficits constitute the same construct, we again conducted a factor analysis using the two ADHD symp-

TABLE 7.3. Correlations of BDEFS Scores with ADHD Symptom Ratings from an Adult ADHD Rating Scale in the Normative Sample

	ADHD symptom scores		
BDEFS scores	Inattentive	Hyp-Imp.	Total ADHD
Self-Management to Time	.74	.46	.67
Self-Organization/Problem Solving	.75	.51	.70
Self-Restraint	.67	.62	.71
Self-Motivation	.70	.51	.67
Self-Regulation of Emotion	.65	.60	.69
BDEFS-LF Total EF Summary Score	.83	.63	.81
ADHD-EF Index	.77	.58	.75
BDEFS-SF Total EF Summary Score	.77	.58	.79

Note. Inattentive = Inattentive dimension score, and Hyp-Imp = Hyperactive–Impulsive dimension score, from an adult ADHD rating scale (Barkley & Murphy, 2006). All Pearson product–moment correlations were significant at p < .001.

tom dimensions with the five BDEFS-LF subscales, and using promax rotation. The results were essentially the same. Once again a single factor emerged, accounting for 68% of the variance. The factor loadings were as follows: ADHD Inattentive = .891, ADHD Hyperactive–Impulsive = .741, Self-Management to Time = .814, Self-Organization/Problem Solving = .843, Self-Restraint = .863, Self-Motivation = .811, and Self-Regulation of Emotion = .823. It is important to notice here that the BDEFS subscale dealing with emotion regulation was available for this analysis, whereas it was not included in the P-BDEFS analyses above. Yet the same results were evident for that new scale as for the others.

These findings replicate the results of our studies of clinical populations, noted above, in showing a substantial relationship between EF deficits in daily life activities and ADHD symptoms—this time in a general population sample of U.S. adults. Ratings of EF deficits on the BDEFS-LF share between 21% and 69% of their variance with the ADHD symptom dimensions, and the highest relationships are with the Total EF Summary Score. Factor analyses indicate that ADHD and EF deficits form a single factorial dimension, thus giving evidence for their representing the same construct. These results also provide evidence of validity for the ADHD-EF Index of the BDEFS-LF in showing significant relationships to actual ADHD ratings in this large normative sample.

This relationship can be better illustrated by selecting from the normative sample those adults likely to have ADHD. As a proxy for diagnosis of ADHD, the Total ADHD Symptom score from the same adult ADHD rating scale (Barkley & Murphy, 2006) was used; a cutoff point at or above the 95th percentile was used for this normative sample. This cutoff point was chosen because of findings that approximately 5% of U.S. adults meet diagnostic criteria for ADHD (see Barkley et al., 2008, Ch. 1; Kessler et al., 2006). The BDEFS-LF subscales for individuals who met this cutoff point were compared to those adults placing at the 84th percentile or lower—a threshold often interpreted as defining the "normal" range, given that it usually equates to 1 *SD* above the mean of a sample. But in defining this group a score equivalent to the 84th percentile was used and not the 1 *SD* threshold because the distribution of ADHD symptoms in a normal population is non-normal and highly skewed to the left (lowest scores). The results for the subscale scores appear in Figure 7.3. All group comparisons were significant at $p < .001$.

The Total EF Summary Score for each group showed the group with adult ADHD ($M = 216.4$, $SD = 44.4$) to be over 3 *SD*s above the distribution of the remaining control sample ($M = 123.1$, $SD = 25.1$), reflecting a markedly high level of EF deficits. Indeed, the mean score for the ADHD group was between the 96th and 98th percentiles for the normative sample on the Total EF Summary Score. The differences in individual BDEFS-LF subscale scores as shown in Figure 7.3 were just as marked. They clearly reflected significant deficiencies in all dimensions of EF in daily activities for the ADHD group. The BDEFS-SF showed an equally impressive difference between these two groups, with the mean of the ADHD-symptomatic group ($M = 48.7$, $SD = 10.5$) being at least 3 *SD*s above that of the control group ($M = 27.3$, $SD = 5.8$) ($F = 733.74$, $p < .001$).

The adults falling into the ADHD range ($M = 26.7$, $SD = 5.9$) on the ADHD symptom scale also showed significant and substantially higher scores on the ADHD-EF Index of the BDEFS-LF than did those in the normative sample control

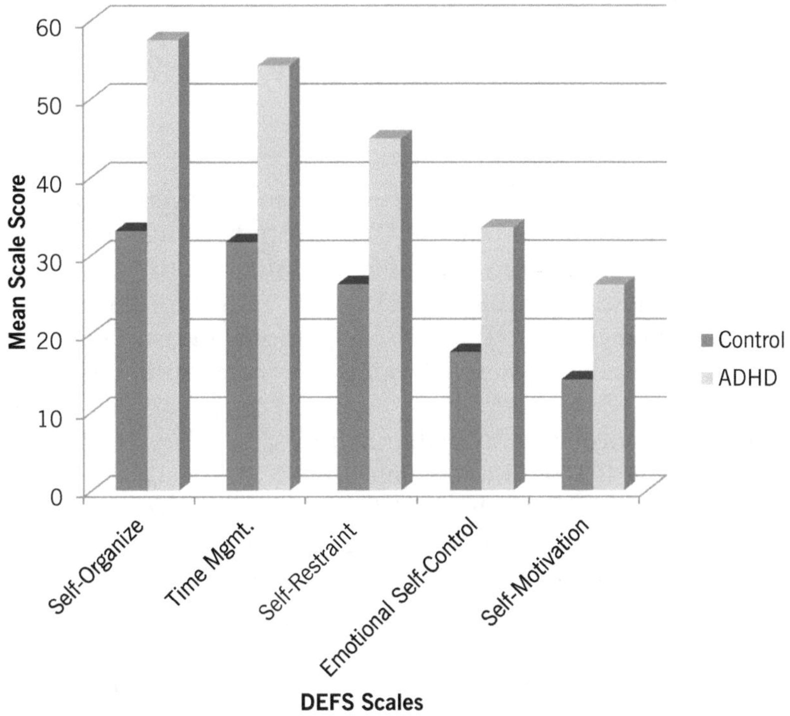

FIGURE 7.3. Comparison of adults with ADHD (defined as scoring at or above the 95th percentile on ADHD symptoms) to control adults (scoring at the 84th percentile or below on ADHD symptoms) on the BDEFS subscales in the normative sample. Self-Organize, Self-Organization/Problem Solving Scale; Time Mgmt., Self-Management to Time subscale; Emotional Self-Control, Self-Regulation of Emotion subscale. All comparisons are significant at $p < .001$. ADHD, $n = 66$; control, $n = 1{,}032$.

group ($M = 15.5$, $SD = 3.4$) ($F = 604.3$, $p < .001$). This again shows minimal overlap in the distributions between these two groups on the ADHD-EF Index. In fact, if a score of 20 on the ADHD-EF Index were chosen as the threshold for identifying adults with ADHD, it would correctly detect 94% of the adults with ADHD (those at or above the 95th percentile on the adult ADHD rating scale in the normative sample) and misclassify as having ADHD just 13% of the control adults (those at or below the 84th percentile on the adult ADHD rating scale). These results also provide more evidence for the validity of the ADHD-EF Index as an identifier of risk for ADHD. And, once more, these findings not only provide evidence of validity for the BDEFS-LF, but also suggest that current theories of ADHD as a disorder of EF are well supported.

Finally, this is an important point to note for future research on the BDEFS with other psychiatric disorders. Evidence may emerge in such studies that psychiatric disorders such as depressive, anxiety, bipolar, conduct, antisocial personality, substance use, or other disorders may differ from control groups in having high scores on the BDEFS. But in view of the strong relationship of EF deficits to ADHD, such studies must control for the comorbidity of ADHD with these other disorders, to evaluate any relationship those disorders may have with EF that are independent of such comorbidity. It is highly possible that some or all of the EF deficits in daily life evident in those disorders are consequences, at least in part, of comorbid ADHD.

Occupational Functioning

We were fortunate to have collected information on the occupational adjustment and functioning of our participants in the UMASS Study, using self-reports, employers' ratings of work performance, and clinicians' ratings on the Social and Occupational Functioning Assessment Scale (SOFAS). The results for the analyses regressing all of the P-BDEFS scales onto these 11 occupational measures after controlling for IQ have been reported elsewhere (Barkley & Murphy, 2010a) and are shown in Table 7.4.

We had similar information available in the Milwaukee Study, in which the interview version of the P-BDEFS was administered and measures of occupational functioning were also collected. The P-BDEFS subscales were correlated with the measures of occupational functioning, and the results, reported elsewhere (Barkley & Fischer, in press), are shown in Table 7.5. We then used multiple-regression analyses to examine which specific P-BDEFS subscales were contributing to the prediction of each occupational measure (Barkley & Fischer, in press). Those results are shown in Table 7.6. These findings from both studies provide evidence for the concurrent validity of the BDEFS in showing a significant relationship between deficits in EF as measured by the P-BDEFS and various measures of occupational functioning assessed from multiple sources in two different studies focusing on adult ADHD.

As with other domains of adaptive functioning discussed below, one cannot draw causal inferences on the direction of effects here between EF and occupational functioning purely from such correlational analyses. Although it may be reasonable to conclude that EF deficits in daily life can clearly interfere with occupational functioning, difficulties in such functioning may also adversely affect self-regulation across time to achieve goals (EF).

Education

If EF in daily life activities is important for educational success and attainment, then measures of EF should show some relationship to the level of education attained by adults. In the UMASS Study (Barkley et al., 2008), we obtained information on the degree of education obtained by the three groups of participants described earlier. For the present manual, correlations were computed between the degree of education and each of the P-BDEFS subscales. Education was negatively correlated with three of the subscales: Self-Organization/Problem Solving ($r = -.132$, $p = .018$), Self-Motivation ($r = -.176$, $p = .002$), and Self-Activation/Concentration ($r = -.122$, $p = .027$). But the relationship with the other subscales was not significant. When the entire sample was sorted into those who had not completed a college degree versus those who had done so, the groups differed significantly on four of the five P-BDEFS subscales and marginally so ($p = .058$) on the fifth (Self-Restraint). Those who completed college had significantly fewer EF problems than did those who had not completed college on these prototype scales. This pattern is illustrated in Figure 7.4 (p. 92).

TABLE 7.4. Predicting Occupational Measures from the P-BDEFS (Self-Ratings) in the UMASS Study

Outcome/predictors	Beta	R	R^2	$R^2\Delta$	F	p
Number of jobs held since high school						
IQ	–.054	.065	.004	.004	1.10	NS
Self-Restraint	.231	.240	.057	.053	14.52	< .001
Self-rated quality of work						
IQ	.032	.063	.004	.004	0.80	NS
Self-Motivation	.366	.370	.137	.133	31.21	< .001
Percent of jobs where person had trouble getting along with others						
IQ	–.094	.109	.012	.012	3.18	NS
Self-Restraint	.363	.379	.143	.131	40.35	< .001
Percent of jobs where person had trouble with own behavior or work performance						
IQ	–.071	.041	.002	.002	0.43	NS
Self-Management to Time	.268	.459	.211	.209	67.33	< .001
Self-Restraint	.227	.475	.225	.014	4.73	.031
Percent of jobs from which person was fired						
IQ	–.092	.059	.004	.004	0.90	NS
Self-Motivation	.250	.255	.065	.061	16.75	< .001
Percent of jobs where person quit due to hostility with employer						
IQ	–.149	.160	.026	.026	6.75	.010
Self-Restraint	.279	.321	.103	.078	22.18	< .001
Percent of jobs where person quit due to boredom						
IQ	–.034	.019	.000	.000	0.09	NS
Self-Motivation	.248	.248	.062	.061	16.64	< .001
Percent of jobs in which person was disciplined for substandard work						
IQ	–.103	.069	.005	.005	1.21	NS
Self-Management to Time	.257	.264	.069	.065	17.82	< .001
Employer-rated impairment score						
IQ	–.054	.036	.001	.001	0.09	NS
Self-Management to Time	.234	.236	.056	.054	4.09	.047
Employer-rated overall work performance						
IQ	–.149	.166	.028	.028	2.45	NS
Self-Motivation	.386	.420	.177	.149	15.38	< .001
Clinician SOFAS rating						
IQ	.121	.095	.009	.009	2.41	NS
Self-Management to Time	–.408	.775	.601	.592	392.37	< .001
Self-Activation/Concentration	–.228	.790	.624	.024	16.72	< .001
Self-Restraint	–.189	.794	.631	.007	4.84	.029

Note. Analyses are for linear multiple regression with forced entry of IQ at Step 1 and stepwise entry of EF scales at Step 2. Beta, standardized beta coefficient; R, regression coefficient; R^2, percent of explained variance accounted for by all variables at this step; $R^2\Delta$ (change), percent of explained variance accounted for by this variable added at this step; F, F to change results; p, probability value for the F-test; NS, not significant. Work performance (both self- and employer-rated) was rated as 1 (excellent) to 5 (very poor). SOFAS, Social and Occupational Functioning Assessment Scale. From Barkley and Murphy (2010a). Copyright 2010 by the National Academy of Neuropsychology. Adapted by permission.

TABLE 7.5. Correlations of P-BDEFS Subscales (Interview Format) with Occupational Measures from the Milwaukee Study

	P-BDEFS subscales				
Occupational measure	S-MT	S-OPS	S-RES	S-MOT	S-ACT
Hollingshead (1975) job index	–.35*	–.29*	–.35*	–.29*	–.33*
Current salary	–.27*	–.27*	–.21*	–.22*	–.18
Self-rated quality of work	.30*	.34*	.29*	.34*	.33*
Average duration of employment	–.08	–.09	–.14	–.08	–.11
Percent of jobs where person had trouble getting along with others	.33*	.43*	.45*	.33*	.39*
Percent of jobs where person had trouble with own behavior or work performance	.41*	.45*	.44*	.42*	.45*
Percent of jobs from which person was fired	.34*	.24*	.32*	.33*	.28*
Percent of jobs where person quit due to hostility with employer	.21*	.15	.30*	.24*	.25*
Percent of jobs where person quit due to boredom	.14	.14	.17	.23*	.13
Percent of jobs in which person was formally reprimanded	.39*	.37*	.44*	.34*	.36*

Note See footnote to Table 7.1 for P-BDEFS subscale abbreviations. Work performance (both self- and employer-rated) was rated as 1 (excellent) to 5 (very poor). From Barkley and Fischer (in press). Copyright by the Taylor and Francis Group. Adapted by permission.
$*p \leq .01$.

We also obtained information about education in the normative sample described in Chapter 3 of this manual. This sample was categorized into four educational levels: less than a high school diploma, graduated from high school, obtained some college education, and completed a bachelor's degree or higher. We compared these four educational groups' scores on the BDEFS-LF and BDEFS-SF via a one-way analysis of variance; the BDEFS-LF results are shown in Table 7.7. The educational groups were found to differ significantly on four of the five subscales and on the Total EF Summary Score. Pairwise comparisons indicated the following rank ordering among the groups in the degree of their EF deficits:

- Self-Organization/Problem Solving: Less than high school > high school > some college, bachelor's degree or higher (the latter two groups did not differ from each other).
- Self-Management to Time: Less than high school education > high school > some college.
- Self-Restraint: Less than high school > high school > some college > bachelor's degree or higher.
- Self-Regulation of Emotion: Less than high school > high school > some college > bachelor's degree or higher.
- Self-Motivation: Less than high school > high school, some college, and bachelor's degree or higher (the latter three groups did not differ from each other).

TABLE 7.6. Prediction of Occupational Impairments from the P-BDEFS Subscales (Interview Format, Self-Reports) in the Milwaukee Study

Outcome/predictors	Beta	R	R^2	$R^2\Delta$	F	p
Hollingshead (1975) job index						
Self-Restraint	–.214	.353	.125	.125	28.88	< .001
Self-Management to Time	–.196	.379	.144	.019	4.49	.035
Current salary						
Self-Organization/Problem Solving		.273	.074	.074	14.86	< .001
Work quality (self-rated)						
Self-Organization/Problem Solving	.208	.342	.117	.117	24.20	< .001
Self-Motivation	.198	.372	.138	.021	4.52	.035
Percent of jobs where person had trouble getting along with others						
Self-Restraint	.282	.446	.199	.199	48.51	< .001
Self-Organization/Problem Solving	.250	.485	.235	.036	9.03	.003
Percent of jobs where person had trouble with own behavior or work performance						
Self-Organization/Problem Solving	.275	.449	.202	.202	48.97	< .001
Self-Restraint	.265	.491	.241	.040	10.14	.002
Percent of jobs from which person was fired						
Self-Management to Time	.339	.339	.115	.115	26.60	< .001
Percent of jobs where person quit due to hostility with boss						
Self-Restraint	.302	.302	.091	.091	20.44	< .001
Percent of jobs where person quit due to boredom						
Self-Motivation	.227	.227	.052	.052	11.17	.001
Percent of jobs in which person was formally reprimanded						
Self-Restraint	.436	.436	.190	.190	48.11	< .001
Employer-rated work performance (age 21)						
Self-Management to Time	.341	.341	.117	.117	20.31	< .001
Employer-rated ADHD severity (age 21)						
Self-Management to Time	.364	.364	.133	.133	23.59	< .001
Employer-rated ODD severity (age 21)						
Self-Restraint	.324	.324	.105	.105	18.03	< .001

Note. Analyses are for linear multiple regression with stepwise entry. See footnote to Table 7.4 for explanation of statistics. From Barkley and Fischer (in press). Copyright by the Taylor and Francis Group. Adapted by permission.

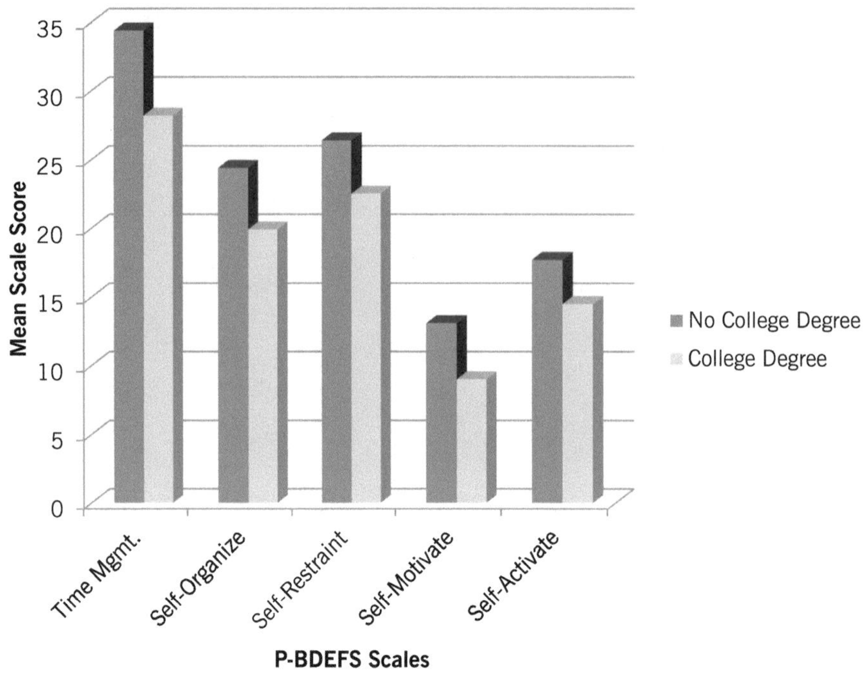

FIGURE 7.4. Comparison of adults with a college degree to those with less than a college degree on the P-BDEFS subscales in the UMASS Study. Data from Barkley, Murphy, and Fischer (2008).

TABLE 7.7. BDEFS-LF Results for Each of Four Levels of Education in the Normative Sample

	Education category									
	< High school		High school		College		Bachelor+			
Score	Mean	*SD*	Mean	*SD*	Mean	*SD*	Mean	*SD*	*F*	*p*
Self-Organize	40.1	15.6	36.2	10.7	36.2	12.0	34.2	10.4	8.82	< .001
Time Mgmt.	35.6	11.8	33.4	10.4	35.0	11.0	34.0	10.5	2.05	NS
Self-Restraint	30.5	10.6	28.2	7.9	29.4	9.2	27.1	6.9	7.51	< .001
Emotion Reg.	20.9	8.3	19.3	6.8	19.8	7.6	18.3	6.2	5.32	.001
Self-Motivation	16.5	6.1	15.1	4.5	15.5	5.2	15.0	4.3	3.48	.015
EF Summary	143.7	44.9	132.3	34.5	136.0	38.4	128.6	32.2	6.46	< .001

Note. Self-Organize, Self-Organization/Problem Solving subscale; Time Mgmt., Self-Management to Time subscale; Emotion Reg., Self-Regulation of Emotion subscale; EF Summary, Total EF Summary Score; *F*, results for the *F*-test from the analysis of variance; *p*, probability value for the *F*-test if ≤ .05; NS, not significant. The four education categories were as follows: < High school, less than high school (n = 136); High school, completed high school (n = 359); College, obtained some college education (n = 357); and Bachelor+, obtained a bachelor's degree or higher (n = 366).

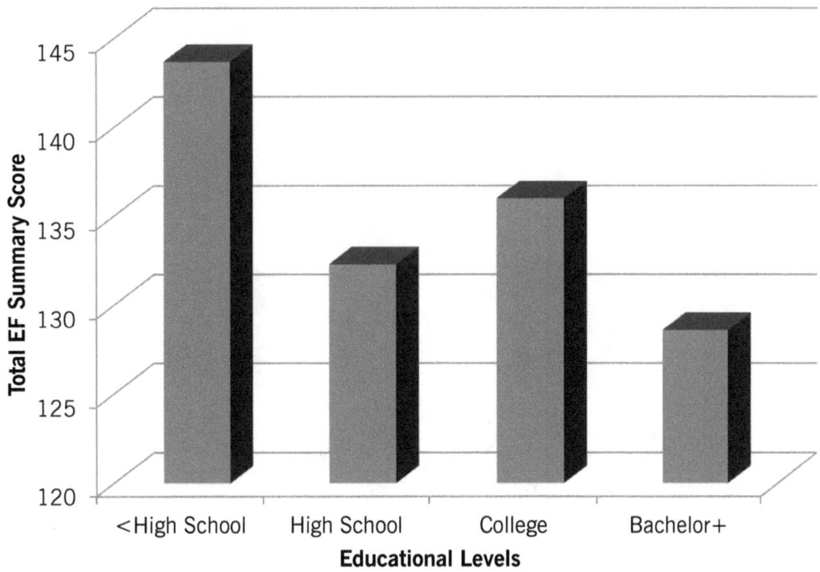

FIGURE 7.5. Relationship of the BDEFS-LF Total EF Summary Score to level of education in the normative sample.

- BDEFS-LF Total EF Summary Score: Less than high school > high school > some college > bachelor's degree or higher.
- ADHD-EF Index: Less than high school > high school > some college > bachelor's degree or higher.
- BDEFS-SF Total EF Summary Score: Less than high school > high school, some college (these two did not differ) > bachelor's degree or higher.

The results for the BDEFS-LF Total EF Summary Score are graphically depicted in Figure 7.5. The overall pattern is consistent with the hypothesis that degree of EF deficits on the BDEFS is associated with obtaining less education, and thus it provides some evidence for construct or criterion validity of the scale. Common sense would clearly indicate that greater problems in EF in daily life ought to contribute to lower educational attainment. Again, however, given that these analyses are merely ones of association and not causation, one cannot infer the direction of influence here purely from these findings.

Employment Status

Of course, it is also conceivable that the degree of EF deficits may be related to adults' employment status, particularly if they are not working as a consequence of disability. The various categories of current employment status in the normative sample were compared on all BDEFS-LF scores and the BDEFS-SF. The results indicated significant differences among the groups on all but the Self-Restraint subscale. For space reasons, I focus here on the BDEFS-LF Total EF Summary Score ($F = 3.26$, $p = .004$); the same pattern was evident on the subscales that were significantly different, as well as on the ADHD-EF Index and the BDEFS-SF. The results

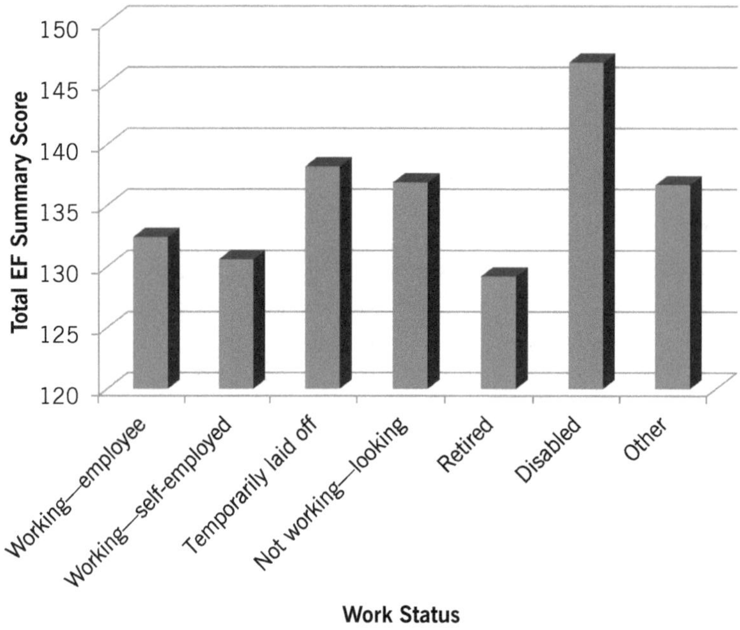

FIGURE 7.6. Relationship of the BDEFS-LF Total EF Summary Score to employment status in the normative sample.

are shown in Figure 7.6. Pairwise comparisons showed that those individuals classified as unemployed due to disability had significantly higher EF problem scores than those in all other categories of employment. The individuals in the other employment categories did not differ from each other in this respect. Clearly, disability status is related to EF deficits in daily life activities and provides further evidence of criterion validity for the BDEFS. Yet, once again, caution should be taken in drawing any causal inferences from these analyses of association concerning the direction of effect.

Household Income

In a similar vein, one can argue that EF deficits in daily life activities would be related to adults' levels of income, particularly since we found that BDEFS scores were related to educational level, and education is known to be related to annual income. Income categories in the normative sample were reclassified into five categories: household income of < \$20,000 (n = 186), \$20,000 to \$39,999 (n = 267), \$40,000 to 74,999 (n = 357), \$75,000 to \$99,999 (n = 282), and \$100,000 and up (n = 126). These income groups were compared on the BDEFS-LF and BDEFS-SF, and significant differences were evident on all but the Self-Management to Time subscale. Again, to save space and because the scores are highly intercorrelated, just the results for the BDEFS-LF Total EF Summary Score are presented (F = 3.50, p = .008). Results indicated that those with household incomes below \$20,000 had significantly higher EF problem scores than those earning at least \$40,000 or higher. The lowest income category also had marginally higher EF problems than those in the next highest category, earning $20,000 to $39,999 ($p$ = .062). The pattern was the same for the BDEFS-LF subscales, the ADHD-EF Index, and the BDEFS-SF, on all of which these groups differed significantly. The results for the BDEFS-LF Total EF Summary Score are graphically illustrated in Figure 7.7 and show overall a decreasing likelihood of EF deficits in daily life with increasing household income. The findings also lend further support to the concurrent (criterion) validity of the BDEFS. And while it is perfectly reasonable to assume that deficits in EF contributed to these differences in financial income, one cannot on the basis of these results rule out the reverse direction of influence—that lower incomes interfere with EF in daily life activities.

Marital Satisfaction and Status

It could also be argued that EF deficits in daily life ought to have an adverse effect on one's marriage. It is not hard to imagine how problems with time management, organization, problem solving, self-restraint, emotional control, and even self-motivation might adversely affect a long-term intimate cohabiting relationship. We found in the UMASS Study that adults with ADHD experienced more marital dissatisfaction (as expressed by both themselves and their partners) than did the Community control adults (Barkley et al., 2008). The relationship of the P-BDEFS to those ratings of marital satisfaction was examined in the UMASS data (Barkley et al., 2008). Ratings of marital satisfaction were made with the Locke–Wallace Marital Adjustment Test (Locke & Wallace, 1959). Consistent with the hypothesis, results indicated that both self-rated and other-rated marital satisfaction were inversely related to degree of difficulties on the P-BDEFS subscales: Self-Management to Time

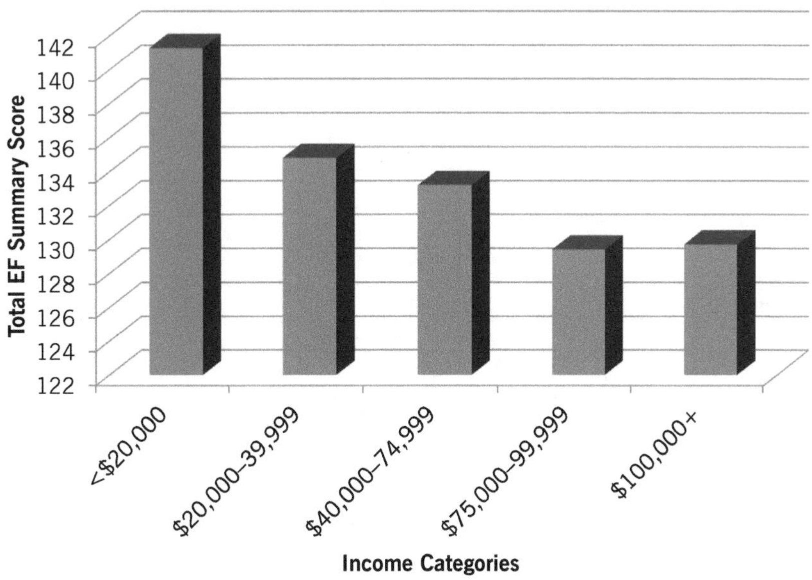

FIGURE 7.7. Relationship of the BDEFS-LF Total EF Summary Score to household income categories in the normative sample.

(*r*'s = –.395 and –.366, respectively), Self-Organization/Problem Solving (–.363 and –.316), Self-Restraint (–.369 and –.351), Self-Motivation (–.425 and –.368), and Self-Activation/Concentration (–.364 and –.277) (all *p*'s < .001).

I studied this issue further in the normative sample reported in this manual, for which information on current marital status was available (see Chapter 3). The various categories of marital status were compared to each other on the BDEFS-LF and BDEFS-SF, using multivariate analysis of variance (MANOVA). Age was used as a covariate in the initial analysis. This was because younger people are less likely to be married and, as shown in Chapter 5, are likely to have higher levels of EF deficits. The overall MANOVA was significant (F = 1.64, p = .023). The subsequent univariate analyses of variance for the BDEFS-LF indicated that the marital groups differed significantly on Self-Organization/Problem Solving (p = .011), Self-Restraint (p = .004), and Self-Motivation (p = .003), as well as on the Total EF Summary Score (p = .009), but not on Self-Management to Time or Self-Regulation of Emotion. Pairwise comparisons for the Total EF Summary Score indicated that those who were married or widowed had significantly lower scores than those who had never married or were currently living with a partner. The results are graphically depicted in Figure 7.8. No other comparisons were significant. This was also the case for the individual BDEFS-LF subscale scores on which group differences were significant, the ADHD-EF Index, and the BDEFS-SF, and so those results are not displayed here.

More research on this issue of the direction of effects between EF and marital functioning/status is clearly warranted. But the results do suggest that a lower degree of problems in EF in daily life is associated with being married, and that high EF scores are associated with lower marital satisfaction. The totality of results here concerning marriage provides still further evidence for the criterion validity of the BDEFS. Do EF deficits in daily life contribute to a poorer marriage or a lower likelihood of being married, or is the direction of influence in the opposite direction? These results cannot give any clear indication one way or the other.

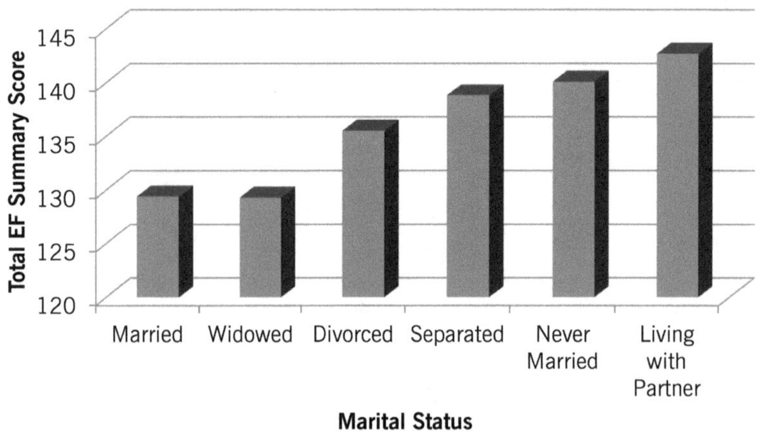

FIGURE 7.8. Relationship of the BDEFS-LF Total EF Summary Score to marital status in the normative sample.

Driving

Researchers have suggested that driving a motor vehicle involves some degree of EF; this may explain the significantly higher problems that adults with ADHD demonstrate in their driving histories (Barkley & Cox, 2007; Barkley et al., 2002). This may be especially the case for such EF domains as self-restraint (inhibition) and self-regulation of emotion, in view of the demands for self-restraint while driving, particularly when one is frustrated by other drivers. The relationship of the P-BDEFS to various self-reported adverse driving outcomes among the UMASS Study adults was therefore examined. Again, emotional self-control was not measured in the P-BDEFS other than by a few items of impulsive emotion that loaded on the Self-Restraint factor, so the full extent to which poor emotional control is related to driving problems could not be examined in this sample. The Pearson product–moment correlations are shown in Table 7.8. All of the subscales as well as the ADHD-EF Index were significantly related to driving risks, and particularly the Self-Restraint subscale, as hypothesized. Again, these correlations may be higher than would be expected in a general population sample, given the overrepresentation of adults with ADHD and adults with other clinical disorders in this study, which would have created a wider range of scores and a higher frequency of adverse outcomes. Even so, the results provide further evidence for the BDEFS in showing some relationship between ratings of EF deficits in daily life activities and impairment in yet another domain of major life activity—that is, driving. As usual, caution is in order here, as such findings do not indicate the direction of influence. But it is certainly more reasonable to assume that EF deficits are interfering with driving than to assume that poor driving creates problems in EF (self-regulation across time). Yet one cannot rule out the possibility that such associations are being driven by yet a third unmeasured variable operating here.

TABLE 7.8. Correlations of P-BDEFS Subscales (Self-Ratings) with Self-Reported Adverse Driving Outcomes from the UMASS Study

	P-BDEFS subscales				
Driving measure	S-MT	S-OPS	S-RES	S-MOT	S-ACT
Number of license revocations	.236**	.152**	.260**	.216**	.171**
Number of vehicular crashes	.124*	.101	.152**	.103	.118*
Number of citations for speeding	.199**	.174**	.214**	.153**	.200**
Number of citations for reckless driving	.174**	.212**	.270**	.199**	.168**
Number of citations for driving under the influence of alcohol	.105	.188**	.212**	.164**	.125*
Number of crashes where person was held to be at fault	.204**	.191**	.265**	.192**	.186**

Note. See footnote to Table 7.1 for P-BDEFS subscale abbreviations. Analyses are Pearson product–moment correlations. *n*'s = 298–328. Data from Barkley, Murphy, and Fischer (2008).
$*p < .05$. $**p \leq .01$.

Credit Rating

Managing money may be still another area of life in which self-regulation across time (EF) and various components of EF (inhibition, planning, problem solving, etc.) may be important in contributing to effectiveness. In the UMASS Study, we obtained participants' self-reports of their credit rating. For the present manual, these credit scores were correlated with the P-BDEFS scores collected in that study, and a significant relationship was found across all subscales. Poor self-rated credit scores were associated with higher problems in Self-Management to Time ($r = .364$), Self-Organization/Problem Solving (.265), Self-Restraint (.274), Self-Motivation (.340), and Self-Activation/Concentration (.244). All correlations were significant at $p < .001$, and sample sizes ranged from 299 to 303. Once more, the P-BDEFS did not assess emotional self-control, and so the contribution of that subscale to the self-reported credit rating was not possible to examine here. And, once again, the direction of influence here cannot be concluded from a correlational analysis such as this. Although it makes perfect sense to assume that deficits in EF (self-regulation) in daily life contribute to problems with financial management, it is also possible that problems with finances feed back to interfere with such self-regulation across time toward goals.

Arrests

Obedience to the law and restraint of antisocial conduct may constitute another domain of major life activity in which it could be reasonably argued that EF may have some influence. The UMASS Study (Barkley et al., 2008) was once again used to study the relationship of P-BDEFS results to the likelihood of having been arrested. The results for the comparison of those who had ever been arrested compared to those who had not on the P-BDEFS subscales are shown in Figure 7.9. All of the comparisons were significant (all p's $< .009$). As hypothesized, higher levels of problems in EF in daily life as assessed by this scale were associated with the likelihood of being arrested. The reason for this association is unclear, and, once more, the causal direction of influence cannot be inferred from such an analysis. It is certainly reasonable, however, to assume that individuals with greater EF deficits in daily life activities have a greater propensity for antisocial conduct and thus are more likely to be arrested, as was evident in the classic case of Phineas Gage over 150 years ago (see Chapter 1).

Health Status

Health maintenance and self-improvement are areas of daily life activities in which EF is also likely to play an important role. Self-Management to Time and its associated foresight concerning the health-related consequences of a person's actions, as well as Self-Restraint and Self-Motivation, may be especially important in adopting and sustaining a healthy lifestyle and altering health behavior patterns that are proving to be unhealthy for the individual. No information on health or drug use was available on the normative sample. But such information was collected in the

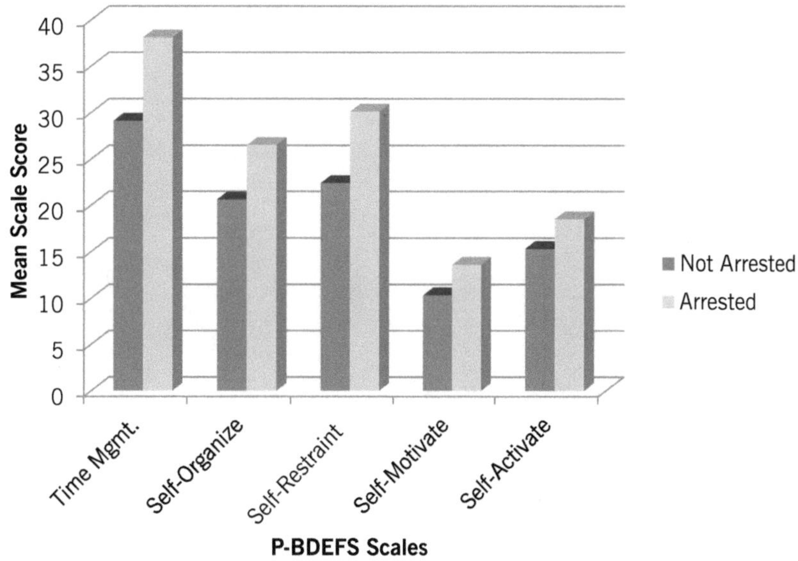

FIGURE 7.9. Comparison of those who had never been arrested to those who had been arrested at least once on P-BDEFS subscales in the UMASS Study. All comparisons are significant ($p < .009$). Data from Barkley, Murphy, and Fischer (2008).

UMASS Study (Barkley et al., 2008), along with the P-BDEFS. Participants in that study who had ever smoked cigarettes (n = 187) were compared to those who did not smoke (n = 131) for the purposes of this manual. The findings appear in Figure 7.10; they clearly show that individuals who had ever smoked had significantly higher problems on all subscales of the P-BDEFS than did those who had never smoked.

We had also collected information from the Skinner Health and Lifestyle Interview (Skinner, 1994), which examined the UMASS participants' lifestyle across 16 domains of health and categorized each domain as being a risk, a concern, or no concern. These domains were nutrition, eating, caffeine use, physical fitness, weight, sleep, social functioning, family functioning, tobacco use, alcohol use, drug use, medication use, vehicle use, sexual functioning, work, and emotional health. These scores were summed across all 16 domains to create an overall Health Index for further examination here. This index was then correlated with the P-BDEFS subscales. The resulting correlations were all significant: Self-Management to Time (r = –.466), Self-Organization/Problem Solving (–.435), Self-Restraint (–.418), Self-Motivation (–.469), and Self-Activation/Concentration (–.429). All correlations were significant at $p < .001$, and sample sizes ranged from 180 to 197. Thus higher EF problem scores were associated with generally lower self-reported health status, as hypothesized. It is important to note once again that although it would be reasonable to assume that EF deficits were contributing to the poor health status of these participants, no direction of influence can be obtained from such correlation analyses. It is just as conceivable that poor health status and lifestyle interfere with EF in daily life activities.

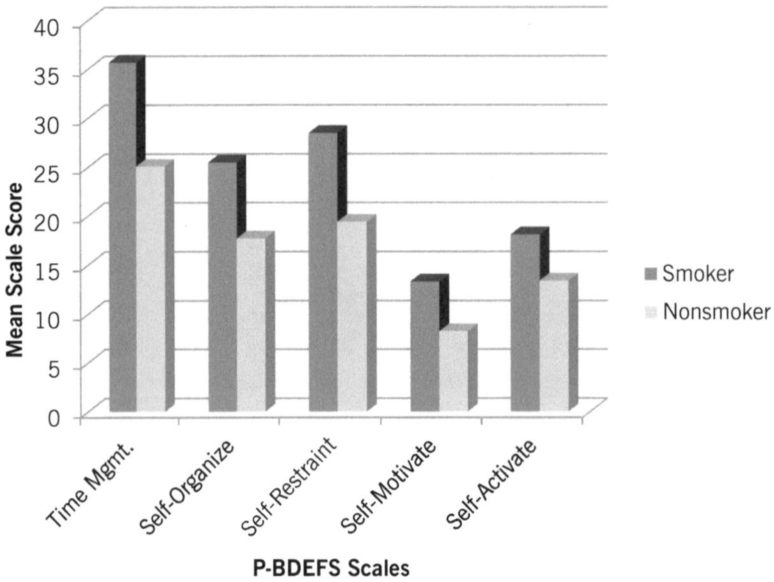

FIGURE 7.10. Comparison of smokers and nonsmokers on P-BDEFS subscales in the UMASS Study. All comparisons are significant ($p < .001$). Data from Barkley, Murphy, and Fischer (2008).

Psychopathology

Various psychiatric and psychological disorders have been associated with difficulties in EF, such as adult ADHD, antisocial personality disorder or conduct disorder (CD), depression, anxiety disorders, bipolar disorders, and autism spectrum disorders, among others. One should therefore find significant associations between the BDEFS and psychological problems of various kinds. To explore this, data from the UMASS Study (Barkley et al., 2008) were once more used to examine the relationship of the P-BDEFS subscales to ratings of psychological problems on the SCL-90-R (Derogatis, 1986). The SCL-90-R provides *T*-scores for nine dimensions of psychological distress: Somatization, Obsessive–Compulsive, Interpersonal Sensitivity, Depression, Anxiety, Hostility, Phobic Anxiety, Paranoid Ideation, and Psychoticism. Once again, we can expect higher-than-typical correlations in this dataset, given that the oversampling of adults with various psychiatric disorders should lead to a wider range and greater frequency of more extreme scores on both measures. Certainly lower levels of association would be expected in a general population sample. The correlations are shown in Table 7.9. They indicate moderate to high relationships between problems with EF in daily life and various dimensions of psychopathology, such that these scales share from 21% to 70% of their variance, as expected. Interestingly, the highest relationships were between the P-BDEFS subscales and the SCL-90-R Obsessive–Compulsive subscale, and to a somewhat lesser degree the SCL-90-R Depression and Anxiety subscales. The adult version of the BRIEF likewise had significant relationships with trait anxiety (*r*'s ranging from .38 to .55 for the State–Trait Anxiety Inventory) and depression (*r*'s ranging from .29 to .59 for the Beck Depression Inventory) (Roth et al., 2005).

TABLE 7.9. Correlations of P-BDEFS Subscales (Self-Ratings) with SCL-90-R Subscales from the UMASS Study

	P-BDEFS subscales				
SCL-90-R subscale	S-MT	S-OPS	S-RES	S-MOT	S-ACT
Somatization	.492	.562	.569	.513	.571
Obsessive–Compulsive	.822	.802	.768	.741	.842
Interpersonal Sensitivity	.701	.734	.744	.686	.746
Depression	.741	.723	.740	.679	.765
Anxiety	.705	.708	.743	.675	.763
Hostility	.651	.662	.760	.669	.751
Phobic Anxiety	.461	.549	.566	.497	.520
Paranoid Ideation	.621	.641	.722	.637	.647
Psychoticism	.639	.687	.687	.624	.697

Note. See footnote to Table 7.1 for P-BDEFS subscale abbreviations. Analyses are Pearson product–moment correlations. (All correlations are significant at $p < .001$.) n's = 295–326. Data from Barkley, Murphy, and Fischer (2008).

Such findings do not necessarily indicate that the P-BDEFS (or BDEFS), or EF rating scales more generally, are contaminated by psychopathology (or vice versa). In other words, it does not mean that the P-BDEFS is just another measure of psychopathology. It is quite reasonable to expect that psychological problems interfere with self-regulation across time to attain one's goals in a social context—that is, with EF as presently defined. It is also reasonable to view that influence as being reciprocal in nature, with EF deficits in daily life exacerbating psychological problems of all types and vice versa.

To show that EF as rated by the P-BDEFS and psychopathology as rated by the SCL-90-R are distinct yet interrelated constructs, factor analysis was used on the subscale scores from both measures. The results appear in Table 7.10. Just two factors emerged after only three iterations in the analysis, and they had eigenvalues greater than 1.00. Factor 1 represents a clear psychopathology factor and has its highest loadings from the SCL-90-R subscales. It accounted for 71.6% of the variance prior to rotation (eigenvalue = 10.0). Factor 2 represents an EF factor and has its highest loadings from the P-BDEFS subscales. It accounted for an additional 8.1% of the variance prior to rotation (eigenvalue = 1.14). The initial analysis was conducted with a varimax rotation, which maximizes the differences between factorial dimensions. After that rotation, Factor 1 explained 41.8% of the variance, and Factor 2 explained 37.9% of the variance. But, as shown above, the two measures were correlated; therefore, the analysis was repeated with a promax rotation, which allows for items to be so correlated. By either approach, the same two-factor structure emerged. Again, the SCL-90-R subscales had their highest loadings on the psychopathology dimension, while the P-BDEFS subscales had their highest loadings on the EF dimension. Yet the two dimensions were clearly interrelated, as discussed above. Especially interesting, once again, is the nearly equal loading of the Obsessive–Compulsive subscale of the SCL-90-R on both dimensions, suggesting

TABLE 7.10. Factor Analysis of the P-BDEFS and SCL-90-R Subscales, Using Varimax (and Promax) Rotations

	Factors and item loadings	
SCL-90-R and P-BDEFS subscales	Factor 1	Factor 2
SCL-90-R Somatization	**.741** **(.784)**	.266 (.544)
SCL-90-R Obsessive–Compulsive	**.665** **(.865)**	.631 (.847)
SCL-90-R Interpersonal Sensitivity	**.797** **(.925)**	.482 (.765)
SCL-90-R Depression	**.754** **(.900)**	.518 (.779)
SCL-90-R Anxiety	**.779** **(.909)**	.482 (.758)
SCL-90-R Hostility	**.667** **(.819)**	.513 (.740)
SCL-90-R Phobic Anxiety	**.804** **(.812)**	.193 (.503)
SCL-90-R Paranoid Ideation	**.799** **(.887)**	.387 (.679)
SCL-90-R Psychoticism	**.796** **(.892)**	.405 (.694)
P-BDEFS Self-Management to Time	.309 (.645)	**.883** **(.932)**
P-BDEFS Self-Organization/ Problem Solving	.419 (.699)	**.772** **(.876)**
P-BDEFS Self-Restraint	.391 (.693)	**.818** **(.906)**
P-BDEFS Self-Motivation	.320 (.644)	**.856** **(.912)**
P-BDEFS Self-Regulation of Emotion	.413 (.722)	**.841** **(.936)**

Note. Numbers in parentheses in each column are factor loadings with a promax rotation. Entries in boldface indicate the factor on which each subscale had higher loadings.

that this form of psychopathology has a strikingly high association with deficits in EF and vice versa. As previously noted about such relationships, however, the direction of influence cannot be gleaned from analyses using correlational methods.

Parenting Stress

A clear and quite reasonable connection can be made between difficulties in adults' self-regulation over time and these adults' parenting ability. Raising children poses significant demands for all dimensions of EF identified on the BDEFS.

We included a measure of parenting stress (the Parenting Stress Index; Abidin, 1995) in the UMASS Study. This permitted the examination here of its relationship to the P-BDEFS. The total parenting stress score from this widely used scale correlated moderately and significantly with all P-BDEFS subscales, as follows: Self-Management to Time (r = .628), Self-Organization/Problem Solving (.674), Self-Restraint (.632), Self-Motivation (.648), and Self-Activation/Concentration (.604). All correlations were significant at $p < .001$, and sample sizes ranged from 49 to 52. The results support the hypothesis that EF deficits in daily life activities have an adverse association with level of distress in childrearing. Yet, again, however, the direction of effect is unclear in such a correlational analysis.

Psychopathology in Offspring

ADHD is a highly heritable disorder. It has been found that the offspring of adults with ADHD are up to eight times more likely to have the disorder (and related disorders, such as oppositional defiant disorder [ODD]) than children of adults in the general population are (see Barkley, 2006; Barkley et al., 2008; Nigg, 2006). Given the strong association of ADHD with problems with EF in daily life activities as discussed above, ratings of EF deficits may well be predictive of this genetic liability in offspring, such that individuals high in EF deficits may have children with a greater risk for symptoms of ADHD and related disorders. This issue was examined here, once again with the UMASS dataset (Barkley et al., 2008). Parents in that study rated their children with regard to DSM-IV symptoms of ADHD, ODD, and CD on the Disruptive Behavior Rating Scale (DBRS; Barkley & Murphy, 2006). They also provided ratings of their children on the Behavior Assessment System for Children (BASC; Reynolds & Kamphaus, 1992), a scale that provides ratings of 12 different dimensions of children's psychological adjustment. The correlations between the P-BDEFS subscales and these symptom severity ratings in the offspring are shown in Table 7.11.

The results indicate a surprising degree of relationship between parental EF deficits and child ADHD and ODD symptoms, and, to a lesser degree, child symptoms of CD. These relationships were of a low (CD) (6–10% shared variance) to moderate (ADHD, ODD) (20–38% shared variance) magnitude of association. It is not clear from such a simple analysis whether the liability here is genetically mediated (parental EF deficits as an index of parental ADHD that confers liability for ADHD in the child), mediated by the family environment, or both. The risk for ODD symptoms is not as surprising as it may first appear, given the recent argument that ADHD involves difficulties with impulsive emotion and that such emotions provide a causal connection to the emotional dyscontrol element of ODD (Barkley, 2010). Likewise, there were low to moderate relationships between the P-BDEFS subscales and all subscales of the BASC. These relationships were relatively higher for BASC subscales evaluating ADHD symptoms than for those evaluating social withdrawal, anxiety, or conduct problems. As before, these relationships were probably inflated by the overrepresentation of ADHD and other clinical disorders in this sample and in these offspring, which would also assure a wider range of scores on both the P-BDEFS and the childhood behavior ratings. Regardless of the mechanism under-

TABLE 7.11. Correlations of P-BDEFS Subscales (Self-Ratings) with Parental Ratings of Child Behavior from the UMASS Study

	P-BDEFS subscales				
Child behavior scale	S-MT	S-OPS	S-RES	S-MOT	S-ACT
DBRS ADHD Inattentive	.624	.523	.515	.564	.561
DBRS ADHD Hyperactive–Impulsive	.534	.492	.458	.516	.503
DBRS ODD	.481	.544	.504	.473	.461
DBRS CD	.259	.293	.385	.322	.307
BASC Hyperactivity	.601	.577	.536	.587	.548
BASC Aggression	.512	.588	.545	.518	.457
BASC Conduct Problems	.411	.501	.485	.498	.369
BASC Anxiety	.579	.416	.586	.488	.555
BASC Depression	.541	.561	.585	.595	.537
BASC Somatic Complaints	.345	.386	.483	.476	.322
BASC Atypicality	.563	.489	.533	.537	.598
BASC Withdrawal	.314	.379	.408	.407	.431
BASC Attention Problems	.617	.506	.508	.573	.515
BASC Adaptability	–.510	–.641	–.605	–.576	–.590
BASC Social Skills	–.313	–.412	–.369	–.445	–.400
BASC Leadership	–.335	–.401	–.399	–.447	–.415

Note. See footnote to Table 7.1 for P-BDEFS subscale abbreviations. DBRS, Disruptive Behavior Rating Scale; BASC, Behavior Assessment System for Children. Analyses are Pearson product–moment correlations. (All correlations are significant at $p < .01$, and most at $p < .001$.) n's = 56–69. Data from Barkley, Murphy, and Fischer (2008).

lying these associations, this is yet more evidence for the criterion (concurrent) validity of the BDEFS. In this case, the BDEFS is indexing a risk for various psychological problems in offspring from parental EF deficits in daily life activities.

Ratings of Impairment in Major Life Activity Domains

We collected various measures of impairment in both our UMASS and Milwaukee Studies. In the UMASS Study, we examined how well the P-BDEFS was associated with a global self-rating of ADHD-related impairment in 10 major life activities (Barkley & Murphy, 2010). We found the following pattern of correlations: Self-Management to Time (r = .83), Self-Organization/Problem Solving (.77), Self-Restraint (.85), Self-Motivation (.77), and Self-Activation/Concentration (.83). Regression analyses showed that three of the P-BDEFS subscales were contributing independently to such impairment, these being (in order) Self-Restraint, Self-Management to Time, and Self-Activation/Concentration. These scales continued to contribute significant variance to the impairment ratings even after we controlled for current severity of ADHD symptoms. A somewhat lower but still impressive pattern of results was found when self-rated P-BDEFS scores were correlated with other ratings of current impairment: Self-Management to Time (r = .70), Self-Organization/Problem Solving (.58), Self-Restraint (.66), Self-Motivation (.62), and Self-Activation/Concentration (.67).

We had similar information available for the ratings of others on the P-BDEFS and their association with the impairment ratings from those others: Self-Management to Time (r = .85), Self-Organization/Problem Solving (.70), Self-Restraint (.87), Self-Motivation (.76), and Self-Activation/Concentration (.84). We also had self-ratings of impairment in childhood (retrospective validity). The correlations between these ratings and the P-BDEFS subscales were as follows: Self-Management to Time (r = .68), Self-Organization/Problem Solving (.72), Self-Restraint (.75), Self-Motivation (.67), and Self-Activation/Concentration (.73). (All p's above were $< .001$.) However, since these ratings were about ADHD-related impairment in various major life activities, and since ADHD severity correlated with P-BDEFS scores, it is not surprising that those same P-BDEFS scores would be highly associated with the impairment ratings. Impairment ratings need to be divorced from ADHD symptoms specifically if they are to be used as an independent measure of impairment.

As part of the data collection for the normative sample, participants completed the Barkley Functional Impairment Scale (BFIS; Barkley, 2011a). This new scale asks respondents to rate on a scale from 0 (not a problem) to 9 (severe problem) how much difficulty they have functioning effectively in each of 15 major life activities. The scale is intended to assess impairment in these life activities *without regard to any specific disorder or psychological or psychiatric problem.* For this manual, the BDEFS scores for the normative sample (N = 1,249) were correlated with each of the ratings of major life activities from the BFIS. The results appear in Table 7.12. All of the correlations were significant and ranged from low to moderate associations. The strongest relationships were evident between BDEFS scores and BFIS ratings of educational activities, managing daily responsibilities, and occupational functioning. This is not surprising, given that these domains are the ones most likely to be placing the heaviest demands on EF (self-regulation across time to achieve goals). These findings provide clear and direct evidence for the criterion (concurrent) validity of the current version of the BDEFS in showing that in a representative sample of the U.S. adult population, higher BDEFS scores are associated with more impairment in every domain of major life activity surveyed by the BFIS and particularly those domains most likely to make the heaviest demands on EF.

Conclusion

In summary, further research is clearly warranted on the reliability, validity, and other psychometric properties of the BDEFS, especially for the newest subscale (Self-Regulation of Emotion, which was not represented in the P-BDEFS). What evidence is available is reasonably broad and substantial, suggesting quite satisfactory validity of the scale. Indeed, there is more evidence for the validity of the BDEFS as marshaled here than for any other rating scale of EF for adults currently available. The evidence is sufficient to support the adoption of the scale for clinical

TABLE 7.12. Correlations of BDEFS Scores (Self-Ratings) with Specific Domains of Impairment from the Barkley Functional Impairment Scale (BFIS) for the Normative Sample

	BDEFS scores						
BFIS domains	S-OPS	S-MT	S-RES	S-REM	S-MOT	EFS[a]	ADHD
In Your Home Life with Immediate Family	.426	.440	.460	.492	.422	.525 (.521)	.482
In Getting Chores Completed at Home and Managing Your Household	.443	.560	.394	.434	.460	.544 (.540)	.522
In Your Work or Occupation	.498	.522	.432	.453	.546	.570 (.566)	.538
In Your Social Interactions with Strangers and Acquaintances	.487	.422	.445	.467	.408	.530 (.524)	.455
In Your Relationships with Friends	.481	.424	.428	.447	.453	.527 (.516)	.464
In Your Activities in the Community (church, clubs, social groups, organizations)	.495	.442	.417	.439	.439	.529 (.522)	.454
In Any Educational Activities (college, night classes, technical training, occupational training)	.575	.548	.476	.471	.559	.607 (.587)	.564
In Your Marital, Co-Living, or Dating Relationships	.449	.475	.387	.376	.395	.459 (.535)	.495
In Your Management of Money, Your Bills, and Your Debts	.354	.441	.387	.376	.395	.459 (.454)	.428
In Driving a Motor Vehicle and in Your History of Citations and Accidents	.354	.306	.368	.328	.386	.402 (.397)	.380
In Your Sexual Activities and Sex Relations with Others	.408	.365	.339	.376	.328	.434 (.424)	.398
In Your Organization and Management of Your Daily Responsibilities	.532	.622	.447	.467	.524	.620 (.614)	.586
In Caring for Yourself Daily (dressing, bathing and hygiene, eating, sleeping, etc.)	.366	.398	.315	.344	.399	.430 (.437)	.411
In Maintaining Your Health (exercise, nutrition, preventive medical and dental care, etc.)	.406	.472	.362	.379	.405	.483 (.483)	.453
In Taking Care of and Raising Your Children	.421	.390	.389	.422	.411	.469 (.470)	.437

Note. S-OPS, Self-Organization/Problem Solving; S-MT, Self-Management to Time; S-RES, Self-Restraint; S-REM, Self-Regulation of Emotion; S-MOT, Self-Motivation; EFS, Total EF Summary Score; ADHD, ADHD-EF Index. BFIS domains were rated on a scale of 0 (not a problem) to 9 (severe problem). Analyses are Pearson product–moment correlations. *n*'s = 875–1,249.

[a]Correlations in parentheses in this column are for the BDEFS-SF Total EF Summary Score.

practice with adult patients, for studying EF in daily activities in research protocols, and for screening adults for EF deficits in daily life activities in industry and other organizations. Scores on the BDEFS or on its earlier and highly similar prototype (the P-BDEFS) are significantly related to difficulties in numerous domains of major life activities. Greater EF problems in daily life on the BDEFS or P-BDEFS are associated with a greater likelihood of impairment or adversity in education, occupational functioning, income, marital relationships, driving, smoking and health status, parenting, psychological morbidity in offspring, and various dimensions of psychopathology, among others.

Research so far suggests that higher problem scores on the BDEFS provide meaningful information about EF in major domains of daily life activities and predictive utility about elevated risks across these domains. To date, evidence indicates that EF ratings, such as those provided by the BDEFS, are far more predictive of impairments in such major life activities as examined here (and probably in others) than is the information provided by far more time-consuming, more costly, and less ecologically valid EF tests or batteries. In determining how well patients, research participants, employees, or others are likely to be functioning in these major domains of adult life, ratings of EF such as those on the BDEFS have proven to be far more useful than have individual EF tests or batteries.

CHAPTER 8

Scoring and Interpretation of the BDEFS Forms

The BDEFS can be used to evaluate EF in daily life activities quickly and inexpensively in a clinical practice, a research setting, or an industrial/organizational setting, among others. It is intended to be used by trained professionals in clinical, research, or industrial/organizational specialties who have sufficient educational background and experience in the evaluation of human psychological functioning and its impairment. Interpretation of the BDEFS subscales, total scores, and profiles requires graduate-level training in a psychological, psychiatric, or medical specialty at an accredited college or university; in particular, it requires training and coursework in the administration and interpretation of psychological measures. Besides carefully reviewing and understanding this manual, examiners using the BDEFS should be familiar with the *Standards for Educational and Psychological Testing* (American Educational Research Association, American Psychological Association, & National Council on Measurement in Education, 1999).

BDEFS Materials

The BDEFS-LF (89 items) is likely to yield more reliable information because of its greater length. But where time is of the essence, the 20-item BDEFS-SF can be used as a quick screen for the likelihood that an individual is exhibiting EF deficits in daily life activities. When clinically significant problems are evident, then a follow-up evaluation can be done with the longer form if an examiner wishes to obtain broader coverage of specific EF domains in such activities. Only the BDEFS-LF yields subscale scores for the five major dimensions of EF problems identified in Chapters 4 and 5: Self-Management to Time, Self-Organization/Problem Solving, Self-Restraint, Self-Motivation, and Self-Regulation of Emotion. Because the BDEFS-SF contains only 20 items, separate scores for each domain are not provided or recommended; only four items are included for each domain, and this is not believed to be sufficient to render a confident evaluation of each domain. A Total EF Summary Score, based on the entire scale's content, is computed for both the BDEFS-LF and BDEFS-SF. And an 11-item ADHD-EF Index can be scored from the BDEFS-LF if a person's risk for adult ADHD is of interest. Finally, the examiner can compute an EF Symptom Count score for each version of the scale; this may be especially informative in clinical settings. A clinically significant symptom of an EF deficit is defined here as any item answered as occurring often (3) or very often (4). This threshold for defining an item as an EF symptom is based on the responses of the normative sample, which indicated that such answers were typically uncommon in that sample (see Chapter 4, Table 4.2).

Two versions of the BDEFS-LF are provided in the Appendix: a Self-Report and an Other-Report form. Norms are only available for the Self-Report version. The Other-Report version is to be collected and scored for comparison to the Self-Report scores, so as to evaluate the degree of disparity between the index person's self-ratings and the ratings of someone who knows the person well. This is discussed later in this chapter. Large disparities should serve as a reason to explore the possible reasons behind them in a follow-up clinical interview with the index person and, if available, the collateral adult.

The BDEFS-LF: Self-Report has 12 score sheets associated with it: one for each sex within each of the four age groups (ages 18–34, 35–49, 50–64, and 65–81), and one each for these age groups where both sexes were combined. Examiners are strongly encouraged not only to plot individuals' scores relative to their sex on the score sheet for that purpose, but also to plot the scores on the score sheet for the entire sample in that age group. The latter score sheet, based on both sexes combined, provides a far larger sample of adults at that age and hence is likely to be more representative of the population at that age group than are the gender-referenced score sheets. Sex differences found in the normative sample were relatively minor and did not occur on all specific domain scores. Where they were present, the sex differences were most apparent at the extreme upper end of the distributions of scores and not at the normal ranges (≤ 75th percentile).

Norms and score sheets are not available as yet for individuals older than 81. What evidence was available for the small group of participants over age 81 in the normative sample suggested that EF deficits had increased in comparison to the earlier age groups. Therefore, the BDEFS-LF and its current norms will need to be used cautiously, if at all, for individuals 82 years of age or older.

Two versions of the BDEFS-SF are also provided in the Appendix, again one for the Self-Report form and a second for the Other-Report form. As with the BDEFS-LF, norms and a score sheet are only available for the Self-Report form of the BDEFS-SF. Again, the Other-Report form is to be evaluated in comparison to the results of the Self-Report form, to determine possible areas of substantial disparity between the index person's self-reports and the ratings of an adult who knows the person well. When such disparities are large, the examiner should evaluate the possible basis for such a disparity through a clinical interview with the index person and, if possible, the collateral adult.

Only a single score sheet is provided for the BDEFS-SF: Self-Report in the Appendix. That is because only the Total EF Summary Score and EF Symptom Count score are computed and then compared to each of the four age groups noted above. The scores are not compared to each sex separately, as for the long form of the BDEFS-LF, because there were no sex differences on either of these scores (see Chapter 5, Table 5.5). Therefore, the scores computed for the BDEFS-SF are compared to the entire sample for each age group, regardless of sex.

Appropriate Purposes and Populations for the BDEFS

The BDEFS forms are not intended to replicate or replace neuropsychological tests of EF. Indeed, the two types of measures are only modestly related if at all, and so neither can replace the other or serve as an alternative means of measuring the same EF components (see Chapter 2). Instead, the extended phenotype of EF (Barkley, 2011a) is best viewed as a hierarchically organized series of levels or as projecting concentric rings outwardly into major human life activities. EF tests and EF ratings are likely to be evaluating quite different levels of this extended phenotype. Therefore, the selection of a measure or set of measures of EF should be based largely on the purpose of the evaluation and the level of EF one wishes to assess. If evaluating the lowest, instrumental, moment-to-moment level of cognitive functioning believed to represent basic EF components is of importance, then EF tests or batteries may be preferred to ratings of EF in daily life. This may be the case in neuroimaging research, in molecular genetics of the instrumental domains of EF, or in the brain localization of specific types of EF. If, however, the purpose of the evaluation is to identify EF at higher levels, of greater behavioral complexity, over longer terms, and in socially significant settings and domains of daily life activities, and to predict the likelihood of impairment in various such activities, then the BDEFS will be of greater utility than EF tests will.

The BDEFS is intended to be used for the evaluation of individuals between 18 and 81 years of age. Typically, these will be individuals who reside in the United States, as this country was the source for the normative sample. Use of the BDEFS with populations, countries, cultures, or ethnic groups outside the United States may be inappropriate, to the extent that such groups vary from the normative reference sample described in this manual.

Administration

The BDEFS-LF: Self-Report or BDEFS-SF: Self-Report should be given directly to the person being asked to complete the rating, along with a clear explanation of the purpose for which the rating is being obtained. The examiner should also make sure the person understands the instructions for completing the rating scale (see these two forms in the Appendix), as well as an opportunity for the individual to express concerns or ask questions about the scale. Although the BDEFS may be mailed out to individuals to complete before the day of the intended evaluation of which the BDEFS is only a part, this should be accompanied with a cover letter that provides information concerning the purpose for which the scale is being used and instructions for its completion. This letter should also contain a means by which the rater can contact the examiner with any concerns or questions about the scale or its intended purpose.

The BDEFS-LF takes an average of 15–20 minutes or less to complete by the average adult in the general population, whereas the BDEFS-SF may take only 4–5 minutes to complete. After the form has been completed, the examiner should review the scale for any missed items and then encourage the rater to complete those items. The failure to complete more than a few items on the scale is likely to invalidate the resulting scores and make the use of the normative tables on the score sheets inappropriate. If the scale has been returned by mail and there is no further opportunity to complete any missed items, these items should be answered with 1 (never or rarely) to create a conservative bias to the scores, so that EF deficits are not unduly exaggerated. Even then, failure to complete more than 5% of the items on the scale should be considered sufficient cause to invalidate the scale (6+ items on the BDEFS-LF, 3+ items on the BDEFS-SF).

Scoring and Interpreting the BDEFS-LF

BDEFS-LF: Self-Report

Follow these procedures to score the BDEFS-LF: Self-Report:

- The easiest method for scoring is to start with Section 1. Add up all of the answers circled in this section. If you prefer, you can add up all of the answers for which 1 (never or rarely) is circled in column 2 of this section (the actual questions are in column 1). Place that sum in the empty box below that column (the box is in the shaded row marked "Office Use Only"). Now do the same for column 3: Sum all of the answers for which 2 (sometimes) is circled in this column, and place that sum at the bottom of that column in the empty box. Repeat this process for columns 4 (answers for which 3 [often] is circled) and column 5 (answers for which 4 [very often] is circled). Now add these four sums together to get the total score for Section 1. Write the answer on the line marked "Section 1 Total Score." This will be in the shaded row at the end of this section.

- Repeat this procedure for Sections 2–5 to get the total score for each of those sections. The section scores correspond to each of the five BDEFS-LF subscales: Section 1, Self-Management to Time; Section 2, Self-Organization/Problem Solving; Section 3, Self-Restraint; Section 4, Self-Motivation; and Section 5, Self-Regulation of Emotion.

- When you have computed each of these section total scores, add them up to get the Total EF Summary Score, which is the total score for the entire scale. Place the answer in the third-from-last row of the scale, marked "Total EF Summary Score" (this row is also shaded and marked "Office Use Only").

• Finally, go back over the entire scale and count the number of items that were answered with a 3 (often) or a 4 (very often) to get the EF Symptom Count. Enter this number in the box so labeled in the next-to-last row of the scale, again marked "Office Use Only."

You have now computed seven scores for the BDEFS-LF: the five subscale total raw scores, the Total EF Summary Score (sum of the five subscale scores), and the EF Symptom Count.

Select the BDEFS-LF Score Sheet for this individual's age group and sex. Each column of this score sheet shows a range of potential raw scores. Start with the column for Self-Management to Time, and circle the score (or score range) in this column that reflects the respondent's score for Section 1 of the BDEFS-LF. Look to the far left column to determine the percentile of the general population that this score represents. The higher the percentile, the more deviant the score is relative to the normative sample (general population). The percentiles that reflect the normal range of deficits are shown as ranges (1–25, 26–50, and 51–75) because scores in these quartiles generally have little clinical significance other than to indicate that an individual's EF in a particular domain is not abnormal. However, scores in the highest quartile begin to take on some clinical significance as indicators of clinical deficiencies and higher associated risks for impairments. For this reason, individual percentiles are provided for each raw score above this threshold. Generally, scores from the 76th to the 84th percentile should be considered of *marginal* clinical significance. Those from the 85th to the 92nd percentile should be considered *borderline or somewhat deficient.* Those between the 93rd and 95th percentiles should be considered *mildly deficient.* Those between the 96th and 98th percentiles should be considered *moderately deficient.* And those at the 99th percentile should be viewed as *markedly deficient or severe.*

Now do the same for the Self-Organization score (the total raw score from Section 2 of the BDEFS-LF: Self-Report); that is, circle the score that represents the respondent's raw score for Section 2. Repeat this procedure for the scores from Sections 3–5 (Self-Restraint, Self-Motivation, and Self-Regulation of Emotion). Then follow the same procedure to get the percentile for the Total EF Summary Score, using that column of the score sheet. In general, the higher the percentile represented by a person's score, the greater the likelihood that this individual may experience some impairment in major daily life activities as a consequence of his or her level of EF deficits.

ADHD-EF Index

If you wish to compute the ADHD-EF Index to evaluate the likelihood that the respondent may have adult ADHD, then add up the scores on the form for the 11 items constituting this index. Each of these 11 items has a shaded box surrounding its item number; the items are 1, 6, 14, 16, 24, 49, 50, 55, 60, 65, and 69. (They are also listed in the last line of the scale.) Place the sum for these items in the last line of the scale, where you see the ADHD-EF Index score indicated.

As a general rule, a score of 20 or higher on the ADHD-EF Index is good for identifying adults with ADHD. It correctly detected 94% of the adults with ADHD (those at or above the 95th percentile on the adult ADHD rating scale we used) in the normative sample, missing just 6% of that group. And it misclassified just 13% of the control group of adults as having probable ADHD (this group consisted of those in the normative sample who fell at or below the 84th percentile on the adult ADHD rating scale). This translates into a positive predictive power (PPP) of 94% and a negative predictive power (NPP) of 87%. PPP refers to the probability that a person will have ADHD, given a score of 20 or higher on this index. NPP refers to the probability that the person will fall into the normal range of ADHD symptoms (i.e., will not have ADHD), given a score of 19 or less on this index.

I must emphasize that the ADHD-EF Index is *not* the sole basis for or a substitute for a clinical evaluation and eventual diagnosis of ADHD in an adult; it is just *an indicator of risk* for adult ADHD. Anyone scoring 20 or above on this index should be considered a candidate for a more thorough clinical evaluation, in order to make (or rule out) a formal diagnosis of adult ADHD and determine any need for treatment. For a more precise determination of the respondent's level of deviation (percentile) from the general population on this index, see the score sheet corresponding to that person's age and sex. Circle the person's score in the column for the ADHD-EF Index, and then look to the far right (last) column for the percentile range in which this would place the person, relative to the general population (normative sample). Typically, as noted earlier, scores at or above the 95th percentile are viewed as clinically significant, while those between the 90th and 94th percentiles should be viewed as being marginally significant and as at least a cause for clinical concern.

EF Symptom Count

You may also wish to obtain a count of the number of items that were answered with a sufficiently high (rare) response as to indicate likely clinical symptoms of an EF deficit. To do so, take the score sheet for the EF Symptom Count. This sheet contains a single table for all age groups. It is not broken down by sex because there were no significant sex differences in the normative sample for this score. Choose the column that corresponds to the person's age group. In that column, find and circle the score (or score range) that corresponds to the raw score you computed for the EF Symptom Count. By looking at the first column at the far left (or the last column at the far right) of this sheet, you will find the percentile (or percentile range) for that score relative to the general population (normative) sample.

BDEFS-LF: Other-Report

The purpose of the BDEFS-LF: Other-Report is to allow clinicians or researchers to obtain the report of an adult who knows a patient or participant well enough to complete the BDEFS-LF concerning that person. The form is scored in the same fashion as the BDEFS-LF: Self-Report (see above). But norms and percentile scores are not available for scoring and interpreting the Other-Report relative to a general population sample. One reason for this is that it is not clear just what such norms would mean in a clinical evaluation. Also, given that the different relationships of informants to the person being rated yield significant differences in results, norms would need to be collected for each type of relationship (parents, siblings/friends, spouses/cohabiting partners) (see Barkley et al., in press). That would be an exceptionally impractical undertaking. Moreover, norms for how people rate each other relative to the general population would seem not to address the more important clinical issue, which is the degree of agreement or disparity between what a specific individual reports about him- or herself and what someone else would report about this person. To achieve that comparison, you should examine the raw scores obtained on both forms for the degree of their disparity or agreement. Some disparity is to be expected. But the greater the disparity, the more reason you would have to inquire further in a clinical interview about the possible reasons for such wide variation. In doing so, you can at least look at the score sheets to see what the percentiles are that correspond to the Other-Report scores, *as if* they were scores from the Self-Report form. Drastic differences in these percentiles would provide another reason to evaluate the basis for such self–other disparities in ratings of EF through interviews with these individuals. What constitutes a clinically significant disparity? See the discussion of score interpretation below for a table that provides such suggested thresholds.

Research on self–other rating disparities in the field of adult ADHD has indicated that spouses/cohabiting partners may be in the best position to provide such reports about current functioning, given the frequency with which they are able to observe the adults with ADHD (Barkley et al., in press). However, the variation in other-reports as a function of a collateral adult's relationship to a patient/participant is relatively minor.

More important appears to be the age of the patient/participant. Younger individuals, particularly below 27 years of age, often report substantially lower levels of symptoms than do those who know them well. In contrast, individuals age 30 or older appear to report higher levels of symptoms than do others who know them well. I am aware of no research on this issue of self–other disparities in EF ratings, or on the relationship of age to such disparities, other than what has been reported for the P-BDEFS in Chapter 7. But given that some researchers consider ADHD symptoms actually to reflect EF deficits, or at least to be highly correlated with them (see Chapter 7), the information about self–other disparities in the field of ADHD may have some bearing on those in the assessment of EF via rating scales. Our research on the P-BDEFS as well as on ADHD ratings has also shown that the degree of disparity is significantly related to the degree of ADHD in both general population and clinical samples. In clinical samples, the levels of anxiety and depression in the index person are also related to the size of the disparity in P-BDEFS ratings. Again, the presence of large disparities in the self–other ratings on the BDEFS-LF should indicate the need to assess whether either of these comorbid disorders is a possible explanation for the disparity.

Scoring the BDEFS-SF

The scoring of the BDEFS-SF: Self-Report is obviously easier than that of the BDEFS-LF, given that only 20 items need to be considered for scoring, compared to the 89 items in the long form.

- First, sum the total for the answers circled in response to Items 1–4. These constitute the Self-Management to Time subscale.
- Place this answer in the last (shaded) row at the end of the scale under "Office Use Only," where you see the blank line for these four items.
- Then do the same for Items 5–8. These represent the Self-Organization subscale.
- Repeat this for Items 9–12 (Self-Restraint), 13–16 (Self-Motivation), and 17–20 (Self-Regulation of Emotion).
- When you have entered all of these scores at the end of the scale, add them all together to obtain the Total EF Summary Score.
- Finally, review the scale responses and count the number of items that were answered with a 3 (often) or a 4 (very often). This is the EF Symptom Count. Enter this where indicated in the last row of the scale.

Use the BDEFS-SF Score Sheet to translate these scores into their respective percentiles based on the normative sample. In this score sheet, you will find two columns for each of the four age groups. The first column under each age group is for the Total EF Summary Score, and the second column is for the EF Symptom Count. These are the only two scores for which norms are provided for this short form. The norms are not broken down by sex because there were no significant sex differences on them in the normative sample, as noted above. Find the columns in that table that correspond to the respondent's age group. Then look down the first of those two columns for the score or range of scores that corresponds to this person's Total EF Summary Score. Circle this score. Look to either the far left or far right column to locate the percentile (or percentile range) that corresponds to that score. Then enter the score for the Total EF Symptom Count in the column to the right that is for this same age group. Again, do this by placing a circle around the raw score that corresponds to the person's raw Total EF Summary Score. Once more, look to the far left or far right column to find the percentile that corresponds to this score relative to the general population for that age group.

The BDEFS-SF: Other-Report form can be used to compute the raw scores to be entered at the bottom on the last line of that scale, just as described above for the Self-Report form. You can then compare these raw scores to those from the Self-Report to evaluate the degree of self–other disparity between the ratings. Once again, as with the BDEFS-LF, sizeable disparities should be a cause for further evaluation through a clinical interview with the index person and, if desired, with the person who completed the Other-Report. As noted above, evidence suggests that severity of ADHD, anxiety, and depression can contribute to such greater-than-typical disparities and should be explored further in the clinical evaluation. The suggested thresholds for these difference scores are provided later in this chapter, to give some rough guidelines as to how large a disparity should be considered unusual or atypical in the general population. As with the BDEFS-LF, you can also look at the score sheet for the BDEFS-SF: Self-Report to see what the equivalent percentiles would be for the various raw scores from the Other-Report. You can do this to see whether those percentiles differ vastly from the ones obtained for the Self-Report. In other words, you can look up the Other-Report percentile scores *as if* these raw scores had been provided on the Self-Report score sheet. Again, dramatic differences between the actual Self-Report percentiles and the hypothetical Other-Report percentiles would be a good reason to explore possible reasons for such marked disparities through further clinical interviewing of these individuals.

The BDEFS–SF Clinical Interview: Self-Report

Very rarely, situations may arise in which an individual being evaluated is unable to complete the BDEFS-LF or BDEFS-SF—perhaps because the person cannot read at all, cannot read English, or has a visual impairment that is sufficiently severe to preclude completing either of these rating scales. In such instances, the examiner may opt to use the BDEFS-SF Clinical Interview: Self-Report, which is an interview version of the BDEFS-SF: Self-Report. Examiners are strongly encouraged to use the BDEFS rating scales whenever possible, as there are no norms that are directly applicable to the Clinical Interview form. But in these rare circumstances, an examiner can use this form to conduct a short interview, in order to determine whether an individual has significant EF deficits in daily life activities.

Instructions to be read to the person being interviewed are provided at the top of the Clinical Interview form. The individual is to be asked whether he or she has experienced each item during the past 6 months often or very often, relative to other individuals of this person's age group. Simply place a check in either the Yes or No column, based on the person's response to each question. After the interview, add up the number of Yes responses to get the EF Symptom Count. Although no norms are available for this interview form, it has been found to be highly correlated with the BDEFS-SF: Self-Report rating scale (.90+). Therefore, to gain a very rough estimate of how deviant the respondent's reports may be, simply look at the column for the EF Symptom Count for the person's age group on the BDEFS-SF: Self-Report score sheet. Then look at the far left or far right column to see the percentile that corresponds to this raw score. It must be emphasized that this provides only a very rough approximation of the individual's status relative to others in the normative population, as the interview form was not given to people in the normative sample. This is why examiners are encouraged to use the rating scale versions of the BDEFS self-report forms whenever possible.

Using the BDEFS to Evaluate Response to Treatment

The BDEFS-LF or BDEFS-SF can be a valuable tool in evaluating an individual's response to various forms of treatment, such as cognitive training as part of neurorehabilitation interventions; cognitive-behavioral treatment of ADHD in adults; or medication treatments, such as the use of ADHD drugs to treat ADHD in an adult. Although the BDEFS-LF can be used for this purpose, the BDEFS-SF provides a less time-consuming and more cost-effective means of doing so.

How much change in a score would be needed to interpret that change as reliable—that is, as being a likely result of the intervention? Scientists and clinicians have employed various methods for determining how much change should be considered as a positive (or negative) response to treatment, such as a change of 20%,

30%, or 40% from the baseline score. But several statistical approaches are better for this purpose because, unlike such arbitrarily defined thresholds for change, these approaches take into consideration the test–retest reliability of the measure and the variation in change scores in the general population. Of these various approaches, one used quite frequently is the "reliable change index" (RCI) developed by Jacobson and colleagues (Jacobson, Roberts, Berns, & McGlinchey, 1999; Jacobson & Truax, 1991). This approach ensures that the degree of change exceeds what may result merely from measurement error or unreliability. In essence, it shows whether the change in the scores from pre- to posttreatment can be assumed, with 95% confidence (probability), to have come from a distribution different from that occurring as a consequence of variation and unreliability alone. A difference in scores of a magnitude at or exceeding the RCI (threshold) would be expected less than 5% of the time by chance and unreliability of measurement alone.

The formula for calculating the RCI is $(X_2 - X_1)/S_{\text{diff}}$, where X_2 is the individual's posttest score and X_1 is the pretest score. The difference between the two is then divided by the standard error of the difference scores (S_{diff}). S_{diff} can be obtained directly from our data by inserting the standard deviations as well as the test–retest reliability information for each scale into the formula provided by Jacobson and Truax (1991). When the difference in means is divided by the S_{diff}, and the resultant number equals or exceeds 1.96, the difference is considered reliable (i.e., it would occur 5% or less of the time by chance alone). But to save you time, the RCI values that would be considered to indicate a significant change on the BDEFS-LF or BDEFS-SF have been calculated for your convenience. Those RCI values are shown in Table 8.1 for each age group. To use them, simply take the posttest score of a patient or participant and subtract it from his or her pretest score. Then look in Table 8.1 in the row that corresponds to which score is being used to evaluate change. Look in the column of that row for the patient's age group. If this change in the patient's scores meets or exceeds the value in this cell of the table, then the change can be considered reliable, or outside the measure's range of error. Probably the best score to use in these cases would be the BDEFS-LF Total EF Summary Score, but the BDEFS-LF subscale scores can also be examined for their reliable change if that is of interest. The use of subscale scores is not recommended for the BDEFS-SF, given that only four items constitute each subscale for this version. If the BDEFS-SF is being used for this purpose, then only the Total EF Summary Score should be used. That is why RCI subscale values are not provided for the BDEFS-SF in Table 8.1.

The fact that a change in scores is reliable does not necessarily make it clinically significant or meaningful, however. One means of establishing such significance is to determine whether the person's score after treatment now falls within the "normal" range of scores following the intervention. For this determination, Jacobson and Truax (1991) have recommended that the posttreatment score should now place within 2 *SD*s of the mean, or the 98th percentile, for the normal population. This is a fairly generous interpretation of "normalization." Others might recommend that the posttreatment score place within 1.5 *SD*s of the normal mean, or approximately the 93rd percentile, since this is a threshold often used to determine whether someone is clinically symptomatic or not. These demarcations for the general population sample for each age group are provided in Table 8.2. Thus, if (1) a patient has shown a change in scores from pretreatment to posttreatment that meets or surpasses the

TABLE 8.1. The Reliable Change Index (RCI) Necessary for Pre- to Posttreatment Difference Scores to Be Significant (Reliable) on the BDEFS-LF Subscales and the BDEFS-LF and BDEFS-SF Total EF Summary Scores

	RCI by age group			
Score	18–34	35–49	50–64	65–81
Self-Management to Time	13.49	13.14	12.23	9.26
Self-Organization/Problem Solving	10.78	11.04	10.61	8.41
Self-Restraint	12.48	11.83	10.27	8.58
Self-Motivation	9.91	8.88	8.20	5.30
Self-Regulation of Emotion	10.40	10.40	8.19	6.77
BDEFS-LF Total EF Summary Score	44.35	44.68	39.91	29.16
BDEFS-SF Total EF Summary Score	11.90	11.90	10.41	7.56

RCI score in Table 8.1, *and* (2) the patient's posttreatment score is within 1.5 or 2 *SD*s of the mean for the normative sample (depending on how lenient the chosen definition of recovery is), one could conclude that the treatment has resulted not only in reliable change but also in recovery or normalization.

As an example, let us consider a male patient with adult ADHD who is 28 years of age and manifesting significant EF deficits in daily life, as reflected in a BDEFS-LF Total EF Summary Score of 260. According to the appropriate BDEFS-LF: Self-Report score sheet in the Appendix for this patient, he is above the 99th percentile of the normative population in the 18–34 age group (either males only or the combined sample of males and females). Following the introduction of treatment for a month with an ADHD medication, the individual completes the BDEFS-LF again and now has a Total EF Summary Score of 180. According to the same score sheet in the Appendix, the patient now places within the 75th- to 84th-percentile range. Is this degree of change from the medication treatment reliable? That is, is it likely to

TABLE 8.2. The Thresholds for Determining Normalization or Recovery at Posttreatment Testing

	Age group							
	18–34		35–49		50–64		65–81	
Score	1.5	2.0	1.5	2.0	1.5	2.0	1.5	2.0
Self-Management to Time	54.4	60.3	50.9	56.7	50.4	55.8	44.3	48.4
Self-Organization/Problem Solving	55.1	61.3	53.6	59.9	54.6	60.7	50.5	55.3
Self-Restraint	44.4	49.2	41.4	46.0	40.4	44.0	37.3	40.6
Self-Motivation	25.2	28.1	23.0	25.6	22.5	24.9	19.0	20.6
Self-Regulation of Emotion	32.5	36.5	31.7	35.7	28.4	31.6	26.0	28.6
BDEFS-LF Total EF Summary Score	200.4	220.4	191.5	211.7	187.9	205.9	167.7	180.9
BDEFS-SF Total EF Summary Score	44.9	49.5	43.0	47.6	42.4	46.6	37.4	40.5

Note. Thresholds are provided for 1.5 and 2 *SD*s above the mean of the normative sample for each age group for the BDEFS-LF subscales and for the BDEFS-LF and BDEFS-SF Total EF Summary Scores.

fall outside the realm of measurement error or unreliability? To find out, let us compute the patient's change score as follows: Pretest score (260) minus posttest score (180) = 80 points. Table 8.1 shows that for 18- to 34-year-olds, the RCI needed to be significant for the Total EF Summary Score is 44.35. The patient's change score of 80 is well above this RCI threshold. Thus the clinician can feel confident that the improvement in the patient's EF deficits is not simply due to measurement error or unreliability and is likely to be a consequence of the treatment. It is reliable. This patient can be considered a treatment responder, assuming that side effects of the medication are not so annoying as to warrant treatment discontinuation.

Next we wish to know whether this patient has been "normalized" by the treatment—that is, whether the intervention has brought him to within the normal range. Table 8.2 shows that the threshold for 2 *SD*s above the normal mean for 18- to 34-year-olds is 220.4, which corresponds to approximately the 98th percentile. The patient's posttest score of 180 is well below this figure, and so could be considered to place within the broadly defined normal range. However, as noted above, some clinicians and researchers believe that this is too generous a definition of "normalization" for determining recovery. Using the criterion of 1.5 *SD*s above the normal mean may be preferred. In that case, the appropriate column of Table 8.2 indicates that this threshold is 200.4. The patient's posttest score of 180 is also below this level. And so even by this more conservative definition of "normalization," this patient can be considered to place within the broadly defined normal range for his age group following treatment. This may be considered "recovery." In fact, according to the means and *SD*s in Table 5.4 (see Chapter 5) for the 18–34 age group, this patient's score is about +1 *SD* above the normal mean (M = 140.4, SD = 40). According to this empirical RCI-based approach to defining "treatment response" and "normalization," the treatment has been successful.

Of course, ADHD medications provide only symptomatic relief in such cases, and only when the medication is taken at therapeutic levels. Therefore, the terms "reliable change" (or "positive response") and "normalization" refer here only to a temporary effect of the medication while in use, and not to a permanent alteration of the patient's functioning in the absence of medication management. Although the BDEFS-LF has been used in this example, it would be more efficient (less time-consuming and more economical) in this case to use the BDEFS-SF and the Total EF Summary Score from that considerably shorter scale.

In addressing both of these questions (reliable change and recovery), it will also be clinically informative to have someone who knows a patient well complete the Other-Report form for the same version of the BDEFS before and after treatment as a check on the validity of the patient's reports. It has been my experience in conducting ADHD medication studies with adults that others who know the patients well may actually detect changes in the patients' functioning earlier than, at lower doses than, or to a greater extent than, the patients do in their self-reports. For this reason, it should become standard practice to compare patients' self-reports with the reports of collateral adults who know the patients well. This should be done both to establish pretreatment status and to determine changes that may be occurring as a function of treatment.

To add further to the utility of such an evaluation of ADHD medication, a clinician may want to have a patient complete the Side Effects Rating Scale (Barkley & Murphy, 2006) both before and after treatment, to ensure that the changes taking place in this domain of daily functioning are in fact consequences of the medication and not merely preexisting conditions that went unexamined prior to the medication trial.

Evaluating Change in EF Due to Brain Injury

A very similar approach can be taken to evaluating whether or not an individual has experienced a significant deterioration in EF in everyday activities following some form of brain injury, whether the origin is a traumatic, infectious, cancerous, or vascular event or some other causal factor. The clinician here may be asking this question: Has a reliable and significant decline in EF in daily life occurred in this patient? The RCI figures in Table 8.1 can be used to determine whether the deterioration in functioning is reliable (i.e., probably outside the realm of measurement error). The patient (let us assume this time that the patient is a woman) can complete the Self-Report form of either the BDEFS-LF or the BDEFS-SF on how she believes she is functioning now. She can then complete it a second time with reference to how well she believes she was functioning prior to the event, assuming that memory for premorbid functioning is not believed to have been adversely affected by this event. Just to be more confident on the matter, the clinician should have someone who knows this patient well complete the Other-Report form for the same version of the BDEFS, as both for the patient's premorbid status and for her current functioning. Then the clinician can compare the patient's premorbid and postmorbid Total EF Summary Scores.

Once again, to get the change score, subtract the postmorbid from the premorbid score; in this case, the result will be negative. Now look in Table 8.1 for the Total EF Summary Score for the patient's age group. If the difference in the patient's scores is higher than the RCI value given in the table, the patient's deterioration in functioning can be considered reliable; that is, the change is probably outside the realm of measurement error or unreliability (i.e., likely to occur 5% or less of the time). The thresholds provided in Table 8.2 for the patient's age group and BDEFS scores can now be used to determine whether this patient now falls outside the normal range; both the 1.5-*SD* and 2-*SD* thresholds (approximately the 93rd and 98th percentiles) can be used. This will enable the clinician to say that the patient's postmorbid score is now more likely to have been drawn from a distribution of individuals with impaired or disordered EF in daily life activities than to have been drawn from the general adult population.

Once again, it will prove clinically useful to do the same comparisons for the Other-Report forms completed by someone who knows this patient well, to see whether similar changes are being reported in the premorbid to postmorbid BDEFS scores. The entries in Tables 8.1 and 8.2 are based only on the Self-Report forms of the BDEFS. Even so, one can still use the Other-Report forms to provide some information on the validity of the changes being seen in such cases, given the satisfactory or reasonable degree of interobserver agreement reported for the P-BDEFS in Chapter 6, as well as for self- and other-ratings of the similar and related domain of ADHD symptoms in a number of previous studies (see Barkley et al., 2008, in press). The Other-Report forms in this case are being used as a check on the validity of the patient's self-reports. The guidelines reported above for determining whether a self–other disparity is substantial enough to be due to more than measurement error can be used in this instance as rough guidelines for just how great a disparity is more than measurement error.

In the present example, the clinician may find that the patient has substantially underreported the changes that have occurred in her EF in daily life activities as a consequence of her injury, relative to the reports of someone who knows her well. This may be because the patient's self-awareness has been so dramatically compromised by the injury that she cannot be considered a valid reporter of her own postmorbid status. Given that self-awareness is a major component of EF (see Chapter 1), such an underreporting of change in self-ratings may well be a consequence of substantial injury to the PFC.

Evaluating Change in EF Due to Psychiatric Disorders or Emotionally Traumatic Events

Events that lead to changes in EF in everyday activities, even those that may be relatively transient, do not always have to originate in some injury to the brain in general or the PFC in particular. The conflating of EF with PFC functioning, and hence of two distinct yet partially coupled levels of analysis (neuropsychological and neurological), can mislead clinicians and others into believing that only injuries to the brain can result in EF deficits in daily life activities. It is just as possible that psychiatric disorders such as ADHD, learning disorders, or autism, which have a developmental origin and are likely to arise from genetically and even environmentally influenced subtle maldevelopment of the brain (as in risk gene × toxin interactions in ADHD), can give rise to such deficits. Indeed, as shown in earlier chapters, ADHD, regardless of its etiology, is highly likely to be associated with EF deficits in daily life activities, even if deficits are less evident on neuropsychological tests of EF. As noted in Chapter 2, this disparity in the results of EF ratings versus EF tests has been found for various neurodevelopmental disorders besides ADHD. In short, the absence of evidence of brain injury in patients manifesting significant EF deficits in daily activities as measured by scales such as the BDEFS does not in any way preclude the possibility that such deficits exist and are legitimate. Evidence of neurological etiology is not a prerequisite for establishing the validity of these deficits.

It is also possible even for individuals with normal brain development to experience episodic EF deficits in daily life activities as a consequence of psychiatric disorders that are not always developmental in origin, such as depression and anxiety. Such disorders may be sufficiently profound to interfere with the adequate or effective utilization of EF in everyday life, even if the neurological system underlying EF is itself uncompromised. The ubiquitous feedback loops and networks known to exist in brain functioning, and especially in the relationship of the PFC to numerous other non-EF systems, make it very possible for disorders that do not originate in the EF system (or in the PFC, for that matter) to have a detrimental effect nonetheless on EF in daily life. Just as not all brain disorders lead to disruption of the EF system or its effective use in daily activities, so all disruptions in EF in such activities do not necessarily have to reside in the brain or specifically in the PFC. Indeed, ratings of EF deficits in daily life activities may be even more sensitive to such detrimental effects of psychiatric disorders, or even to the transient effects of psychologically or emotionally traumatic events, than are EF tests.

The existence of deficits at one level of EF is not necessarily contingent on deficits' being found at lower levels in the hierarchy of EF, as discussed elsewhere (Barkley, 2011a). They can arise at higher levels of EF through various non-neurological influences. Likewise, the existence of deficits at a lower level of EF does not automatically ensure their expression at a higher level, given that phenotypic expression at that higher level can be dependent on or moderated by the existence of compensatory external structures or environmental factors at that higher level. The long-standing one-level (instrumental cognitive), one-origin (the brain/PFC) perspective of EF deficits is a gross oversimplification. It is also an erroneous one—not only in view of the accumulating evidence for the hierarchical organization of EF, but also in view of the extended phenotypic effects of EF at a distance, which can be expressed in the expanding spheres of individual daily adaptive functioning, interpersonal social relations, and effective performance in most domains of major life activities over weeks, months, or years.

The cognitive level of EF and its underlying linkage to the PFC did not arise in the course of human evolution to enable humans to take simplistic and socially neutered EF tests. It was most likely selected, in view of the adaptive problems that arose in daily activities most often involving other self-regulating human competitors and cooperators, as a means of addressing these adaptive problems (Barkley, 2001). Ratings of EF in daily life activities are more likely to detect such extended phenotypic effects than are EF tests or batteries of such tests, given their far wider ascertainment window (months vs. minutes), reliance on multiple sources (self and others), capacity to capture more environmental settings and activity domains, greater ability to incorporate the social nature of EF, and capacity to assess more hierarchically complex and temporally extended EF activities than will ever be the case for EF tests. As a consequence, more EF deficits in daily life are likely to be found across more neurological and psychiatric disorders, or even more psychologically compromising situations, than have heretofore been documented by using EF tests.

This easily explains the situation that has arisen in the clinical assessment of EF, wherein examiners have been more likely to document EF deficits in various neurological and non-neurological disorders with EF ratings than with EF tests. Such findings are not cause for frustration with the EF ratings or evidence against the ratings, as if they falsely overdocument EF deficits that do not otherwise exist. They are just as easily seen as evidence that EF cognitive tests are grossly undersensitive to the extended phenotypic expression of EF into important daily activities, over long spans of time, in important domains of human adaptive functioning. And such findings for EF ratings also provide evidence that even non-neurological disorders or transient psychological events may influence the expression or effective utilization of EF in everyday activities, even if the underlying neurological system that gives rise to EF is itself intact.

To reiterate, EF is a neuropsychological construct that does not depend for its existence and utility on some obsessively slavish linkage to a lower biological level of analysis (brain damage) or to some consensus-ordained lab test(s) heralded as the sine qua non of EF assessment. It can be studied for its utility and contribution to understanding human behavior and affairs in its own right, independent of the field of neurology. We can do so provided that EF is operationally defined at its own psychological level of analysis, and that theoretical models of it at that level are testable as well as scientifically and clinically useful. By these criteria, EF ratings (and other observational methodologies) may play a more valuable role than EF tests do in such conceptualizations, model building, and model testing, as well as in the clinical and scientific evaluation of EF. The evidence available, as well as the level of analysis and extended phenotypic domain of interest to the examiner, should be what determines the best means for assessing EF—not some dogmatic adherence to a historically dated obsession with laboratory testing as the gold standard for the evaluation of EF.

Interpreting the BDEFS

A competent professional interpretation of the results of the BDEFS begins with a thorough understanding of the nature of EF and its component dimensions. Although Chapter 1 can serve as an introduction to this topic, it is not a substitute for a more thorough grounding in the larger literature on EF. It is therefore essential for examiners to have not only a thorough understanding of the earlier chapters of this manual, but also familiarity with the neuropsychological literature on EF, especially as it is manifested in daily life activities.

In brief, the BDEFS is intended to measure an individual's capacity to engage in self-regulation across time for the attainment of future goals, especially in social contexts. Specifically, the BDEFS evaluates those neuropsychological abilities that serve to support and contribute to this cross-temporal, future-oriented self-regulation: Self-Management to Time, Self-Organization/Problem Solving, Self-Restraint (Inhibition), Self-Motivation, and Self-Regulation of Emotions. Some interpretive information has been given above in the discussion of how to score the BDEFS. Further interpretation of the scale is based on the following approaches to understanding the meaning of the scores.

Face Validity

The face validity approach to interpretation is aided by a complete familiarity with the items contained in the BDEFS and the five sections (subscales) to which those items have been assigned. High scores on a subscale (typically at or above the 93rd percentile, and especially at or above the 98th) may signal a deficiency in this area of EF in daily life activities. One initial means of interpreting each subscale in a clinical report is on the basis of its face validity. That is, the examiner can actually interpret the meaning of a subscale score from the name given to that subscale (Self-Management to Time, Self-Organization/Problem Solving, etc.). This interpretation can be enhanced by selecting the individual items from that subscale to which the person has responded with a 3 or 4 (these are considered symptoms), and directly quoting these items in the portion of the report that covers the meaning of this subscale. Given that the subscales are moderately to highly intercorrelated, it is most unlikely that an individual will produce deviant scores on just one or two subscales of the BDEFS. Although this is not an impossible occurrence, it would certainly be cause for further exploration of the reason for such an unusual event. One possibility may be a very discrete, focal brain lesion in a small area of the PFC or cerebellum. Another may be malingering. Also in view of this interrelatedness of the subscales, computing interscale differences is not encouraged, as the meaning of such disparities has not been explored in any research to date. This does not mean, however, that relative fluctuations across the subscales will not be evident—only that interpreting the meaning of large disparities among them has no empirical basis at this time. Just interpreting the meaning of each subscale separately is likely to be sufficient to convey the meaning of the BDEFS scores, rather than trying to milk further information out of subsequent comparisons between the subscales for which no guidance can be given here.

Normative Comparisons

Further interpretation of each subscale or other score continues with the comparison of the individual's score to that of the normative population, using the score sheets and the percentiles obtained for them. This is then reported as the relative position of the individual in comparison to the general population of adults, and specifically to the person's sex and age group and the norms used to obtain the percentile score. When the percentile score is used, the individual is said to place at or above this percentage of individuals in the general population of his or her age group (and sex, if the sex-referenced score sheets in the Appendix are used) in EF in daily life activities.

Self–Other Comparisons

Once again, the examiner is strongly encouraged to have someone who knows the participant well complete an Other-Report form, so as to obtain information on interobserver agreement and a quick check on the likely validity of the self-ratings. Interpretation of the BDEFS can then continue with a discussion of the results of this comparison. Care must be taken not to assume automatically that the ratings on the Other-Report form are somehow more valid or should serve as the standard of "truth" against which to judge the participant's self-ratings. This is a relative comparison between two observers, neither of whom has an exclusive claim to the truth. Yet the comparison itself is informative in showing whether one party reports substantially higher or lower numbers of EF problems than the other does. If these disparities exceed the suggested cutoff points given below, the examiner needs to use this as an opportunity to explore possible reasons for these disparities. As noted above, it is not uncommon for individuals below 30 years of age to underreport their difficulties, whereas those over 30 may overreport them relative to the reports of their significant others. Also, recall from earlier in this chapter that comorbidities for ADHD, anxiety, and depression have been found to be associated with greater disparities in self–other ratings and should be explored further in the clinical evaluation. This is especially so for anxiety and depression in clinic-referred populations; in the general population, ADHD is the principal correlate of such disparities.

When should a disparity be viewed as clinically significant or suspicious? In my opinion, the same statistical formula used above in determining the RCI for the change scores obtained from pretreatment to posttreatment evaluations can also be used fruitfully for determining when a disparity between self- and other-ratings is large enough to be considered a reliable difference. After all, in each of these two instances, two scores about an individual from two distinct ratings are being compared; in one the comparison is of two ratings by the same source over time, while in the other it is of two ratings by different sources at the same time point. In either case, the correlation between the two assessments is used to determine whether the difference is reliable. In the first case (pre- to posttreatment scores), the correlation is the one for test–retest reliability and is considered the RCI. In the second case (self- vs. other-ratings), the correlation is the one for interrater agreement and is considered the "reliable difference index," or RDI.

Table 8.3 provides the RDI thresholds for the scores obtained for both the BDEFS-LF and BDEFS-SF. The standard deviations used to create these thresholds were those reported in Chapter 5 for each score for each age group in the normative sample, as they appear in Table 5.4 for the scores from the BDEFS-LF. The standard deviations in Table 5.5 for the Total EF Summary Score from the BDEFS-SF were used to compute the threshold (RDI) for that score in Table 8.3. The interrater reliability correlations used to create this table come from those obtained from the prototype of the BDEFS, the P-BDEFS, as reported in Chapter 6. Since there was no Self-Regulation of Emotion subscale on the P-BDEFS, the average of the interrater correlations for the other four scales (.72) was used to estimate the interrater correlation for this subscale. Because there was no short form of the P-BDEFS, the interrater correlation used for the Total EF Summary Score of the BDEFS-SF was the same as that used for the Total EF Summary Score of the BDEFS-LF (.78).

To use this table, first subtract the other-rating from the self-rating. With this difference score in mind, look in Table 8.3 along the appropriate row for that score and under the column for the index person's age group. The number in this cell is the RDI, or the threshold that this difference score needs to match or exceed to be considered a reliable difference. It is considered a reliable or significant difference,

TABLE 8.3. The Reliable Difference Index (RDI) Necessary for Difference Scores between Self-Ratings and Other-Ratings to Be Significant (Reliable) on the BDEFS-LF Subscales and the BDEFS-LF and BDEFS-SF Total EF Summary Scores

	RDI by age group			
Score	18–34	35–49	50–64	65–81
Self-Management to Time	15.0	14.6	13.6	10.3
Self-Organization/Problem Solving	19.9	20.4	19.6	15.5
Self-Restraint	13.6	12.9	11.2	9.3
Self-Motivation	8.9	8.0	7.4	4.8
Self-Regulation of Emotion	11.7	11.7	9.2	7.6
BDEFS-LF Total EF Summary Score	52.0	52.4	46.8	34.2
BDEFS-SF Total EF Summary Score	12.0	12.0	10.9	7.9

as it would have occurred in 5% or fewer cases. Clinicians should understand that these thresholds in Table 8.3 are relatively rough or approximate guidelines for determining when a self–other disparity in ratings is of such a magnitude as to be unlikely to be due to chance or unreliability of the rating scale alone.

Risk Analysis (Using the Evidence on Criterion Validity)

As discussed in Chapter 7, high scores on the BDEFS or P-BDEFS were associated in our research with various difficulties in various domains of major life activities. Therefore, the higher the scores observed on the BDEFS, the more likely a participant is to be at risk for problems in these same domains. These risks should be noted in the clinical interpretation of the larger meaning of the BDEFS scores, beyond their simply reflecting the five dimensions of EF in daily life for which the subscales are named. Problems with educational and occupational functioning, marital or cohabiting satisfaction, income and financial management, adverse driving outcomes, various forms of psychological distress (anxiety, depression, hostility, etc.), parenting stress, and psychological problems in offspring are all correlates of higher BDEFS scores that deserve notice by the examiner and probably should be conveyed to the participant when appropriate and applicable. Such information can also be linked to what is already known about the participant from the larger clinical evaluation, in which the BDEFS should serve as simply one component. The examiner will have information on the individual's history with regard to these and other major domains of life activity, and the BDEFS findings can be placed in this larger context. The BDEFS results can perhaps provide additional hypotheses or even explanations as to why adverse events in these various domains may have been consequences of or at least associated with deficits in EF. This risk analysis concerning impairments can be further aided by using the BFIS (Barkley, 2011a), on which national norms are available for self-ratings of potential impairment in 15 major domains of life activities. The BFIS also has an Other-Report form, which can contribute further to the evaluation of impairment risk in the patient.

Pre- to Postinjury Status

As already noted above, another approach to interpreting the BDEFS exists when the scale has been used to assess possible changes in an individual after a neurological injury, or in conjunction with the onset of an acute adverse psychiatric or psychological event. If the BDEFS was given twice to an individual (and to a significant other) with instructions to complete one version for preinjury status and the other for postinjury, then these comparisons can be interpreted (with appropriate caution) for the information they may provide about the impact of the injury or event on EF deficits in daily life activities.

Pre- to Posttreatment Change

As discussed above, examiners can also use the BDEFS to evaluate possible response to intervention by giving the scale before and after an intervention has been implemented. Guidelines are given above and in Tables 8.1 and 8.2 for how to interpret a change in scores as reflecting (1) reliable change and (2) recovery or normalization. This information can be included in the interpretation of the meaning of the BDEFS scores so obtained.

Conclusion

The BDEFS provides a clinically informative means of evaluating EF deficits in daily life activities as reported by adults ages 18–81 and by others who know them well (on its Self-Report and Other-Report forms, respectively). Both the comprehensive 89-item form (the BDEFS-LF) and the 20-item version (the BDEFS-SF) can serve to evaluate EF deficits in everyday activities along five interrelated dimensions: Self-Management to Time, Self-Organization/Problem Solving, Self-Restraint, Self-Motivation, and Self-Regulation of Emotion. Further research on and clinical experience with the BDEFS is strongly encouraged. Meanwhile, the evidence obtained to date shows the BDEFS to be reasonably reliable, valid, and useful in assessing these dimensions of EF in daily life activities. It is efficient and cost-effective, while also yielding valuable information on the potential risks that EF deficits may be posing—that is, the extent to which they may relate to potential impairments in various domains of major life activities. The adaptive meaningfulness of the BDEFS is documented in its association with impairment in many such domains, beyond simply documenting the existence of EF deficits. The scale can be used in clinical practice, research, industrial/organizational settings, or any venue where the evaluation of potential EF deficits in daily activities is of interest. It can also serve as a basis for evaluating change in such deficits, whether as a consequence of treatment or secondary to the occurrence of various neurological and psychiatric disorders or even transient psychological events. I hope that you, my readers, find these scales useful in your practice.

APPENDIX

BDEFS Forms and Score Sheets

BDEFS-LF: Self-Report

Name: ______________________ Date: ______________

Sex: (Circle one) Male Female Age: ______________

Instructions

How often do you experience each of these problems? Please circle the number next to each item that best describes your behavior **DURING THE PAST 6 MONTHS**. Please ignore the sections marked "Office Use Only."

Section 1 Items		Never or rarely	Some- times	Often	Very often
1.	Procrastinate or put off doing things until the last minute	1	2	3	4
2.	Poor sense of time	1	2	3	4
3.	Waste or mismanage my time	1	2	3	4
4.	Not prepared on time for work or assigned tasks	1	2	3	4
5.	Fail to meet deadlines for assignments	1	2	3	4
6.	Have trouble planning ahead or preparing for upcoming events	1	2	3	4
7.	Forget to do things I am supposed to do	1	2	3	4
8.	Can't seem to accomplish the goals I set for myself	1	2	3	4
9.	Late for work or scheduled appointments	1	2	3	4
10.	Can't seem to hold in mind things I need to remember to do	1	2	3	4
11.	Can't seem to get things done unless there is an immediate deadline	1	2	3	4
12.	Have difficulty judging how much time it will take to do something or get somewhere	1	2	3	4
13.	Have trouble motivating myself to start work	1	2	3	4
14.	Have difficulty motivating myself to stick with my work and get it done	1	2	3	4
15.	Not motivated to prepare in advance for things I know I am supposed to do	1	2	3	4
16.	Have trouble completing one activity before starting into a new one	1	2	3	4
17.	Have trouble doing what I tell myself to do	1	2	3	4
18.	Difficulties following through on promises or commitments I may make to others	1	2	3	4
19.	Lack self-discipline	1	2	3	4
20.	Have difficulty arranging or doing my work by its priority or importance; can't "prioritize" well	1	2	3	4
21.	Find it hard to get started or get going on things I need to get done	1	2	3	4
Office Use Only—**Section 1 Total Score** ________					

(cont.)

Section 2 Items	Never or rarely	Some-times	Often	Very often
22. I do not seem to anticipate the future as much or as well as others	1	2	3	4
23. Can't seem to remember what I previously heard or read about	1	2	3	4
24. I have trouble organizing my thoughts	1	2	3	4
25. When I am shown something complicated to do, I cannot keep the information in mind so as to imitate or do it correctly	1	2	3	4
26. I have trouble considering various options for doing things and weighing their consequences	1	2	3	4
27. Have difficulties saying what I want to say	1	2	3	4
28. Unable to come up with or invent as many solutions to problems as others seem to do	1	2	3	4
29. Find myself at a loss for words when I want to explain something to others	1	2	3	4
30. Have trouble putting my thoughts down in writing as well or as quickly as others	1	2	3	4
31. Feel I am not as creative or inventive as others of my level of intelligence	1	2	3	4
32. In trying to accomplish goals or assignments, I find I am not able to think of as many ways of doing things as others	1	2	3	4
33. Have trouble learning new or complex activities as well as others	1	2	3	4
34. Have difficulty explaining things in their proper order or sequence	1	2	3	4
35. Can't seem to get to the point of my explanations as quickly as others	1	2	3	4
36. Have trouble doing things in their proper order or sequence	1	2	3	4
37. Unable to "think on my feet" or respond as effectively as others to unexpected events	1	2	3	4
38. I am slower than others at solving problems I encounter in my daily life	1	2	3	4
39. Easily distracted by irrelevant events or thoughts when I must concentrate on something	1	2	3	4
40. Not able to comprehend what I read as well as I should be able to do; have to reread material to get its meaning	1	2	3	4
41. Cannot focus my attention on tasks or work as well as others	1	2	3	4
42. Easily confused	1	2	3	4
43. Can't seem to sustain my concentration on reading, paperwork, lectures, or work	1	2	3	4
44. Find it hard to focus on what is important from what is not important when I do things	1	2	3	4
45. I don't seem to process information as quickly or as accurately as others	1	2	3	4
Office Use Only—**Section 2 Total Score** ________				

(cont.)

Section 3 Items	Never or rarely	Some-times	Often	Very often
46. Find it difficult to tolerate waiting; impatient	1	2	3	4
47. Make decisions impulsively	1	2	3	4
48. Unable to inhibit my reactions or responses to events or others	1	2	3	4
49. Have difficulty stopping my activities or behavior when I should do so	1	2	3	4
50. Have difficulty changing my behavior when I am given feedback about my mistakes	1	2	3	4
51. Make impulsive comments to others	1	2	3	4
52. Likely to do things without considering the consequences for doing them	1	2	3	4
53. Change my plans at the last minute on a whim or last minute impulse	1	2	3	4
54. Fail to consider past relevant events or past personal experiences before responding to situations (I act without thinking)	1	2	3	4
55. Not aware of things I say or do	1	2	3	4
56. Have difficulty being objective about things that affect me	1	2	3	4
57. Find it hard to take other people's perspectives about a problem or situation	1	2	3	4
58. Don't think about or talk things over with myself before doing something	1	2	3	4
59. Trouble following the rules in a situation	1	2	3	4
60. More likely to drive a motor vehicle much faster than others (Excessive speeding)	1	2	3	4
61. Have a low tolerance for frustrating situations	1	2	3	4
62. Cannot inhibit my emotions as well as others	1	2	3	4
63. I don't look ahead and think about what the future outcomes will be before I do something (I don't use my foresight)	1	2	3	4
64. I engage in risk taking activities more than others are likely to do	1	2	3	4
Office Use Only—**Section 3 Total Score** ________				
Section 4 Items	Never or rarely	Some-times	Often	Very often
65. Likely to take short cuts in my work and not do all that I am supposed to do	1	2	3	4
66. Likely to skip out on work early if my work is boring to do	1	2	3	4
67. Do not put as much effort into my work as I should or than others are able to do	1	2	3	4
68. Others tell me I am lazy or unmotivated	1	2	3	4
69. Have to depend on others to help me get my work done	1	2	3	4

(cont.)

70. Things must have an immediate payoff for me or I do not seem to get them done	1	2	3	4
71. Have difficulty resisting the urge to do something fun or more interesting when I am supposed to be working	1	2	3	4
72. Inconsistent in the quality or quantity of my work performance	1	2	3	4
73. Unable to work as well as others without supervision or frequent instruction	1	2	3	4
74. I do not have the willpower or determination that others seem to have	1	2	3	4
75. I am not able to work toward longer term or delayed rewards as well as others	1	2	3	4
76. I cannot resist doing things that produce immediate rewards even if they are not good for me in the long run	1	2	3	4
Office Use Only—**Section 4 Total Score** ________				
Section 5 Items	Never or rarely	Sometimes	Often	Very often
77. Quick to get angry or become upset	1	2	3	4
78. Overreact emotionally	1	2	3	4
79. Easily excitable	1	2	3	4
80. Unable to inhibit showing strong negative or positive emotions	1	2	3	4
81. Have trouble calming myself down once I am emotionally upset	1	2	3	4
82. Cannot seem to regain emotional control and become more reasonable once I am emotional	1	2	3	4
83. Cannot seem to distract myself away from whatever is upsetting me emotionally to help calm me down. I can't refocus my mind to a more positive framework.	1	2	3	4
84. Unable to manage my emotions in order to accomplish my goals successfully or get along well with others	1	2	3	4
85. I remain emotional or upset longer than others	1	2	3	4
86. I find it difficult to walk away from emotionally upsetting encounters with others or leave situations in which I have become very emotional	1	2	3	4
87. I cannot rechannel or redirect my emotions into more positive ways or outlets when I get upset	1	2	3	4
88. I am not able to evaluate an emotionally upsetting event more objectively	1	2	3	4
89. I cannot redefine negative events into more positive viewpoints when I feel strong emotions	1	2	3	4
Office Use Only—**Section 5 Total Score** ________				

(cont.)

Office Use Only **Total of Sections 1–5: Total EF Summary Score___________**				
Office Use Only **Count number of items answered 3 or 4** **EF Symptom Count___________**				
Office Use Only **Add Items 1, 6, 14, 16, 24, 49, 50, 55, 60, 65, and 69** **ADHD-EF Index Score**				

BDEFS-LF: Other-Report

Name of person to be rated: ______________________ Date: ______________

Your name: ____

Your relationship to person being rated: (Circle one)

Mother Father Brother/sister Spouse/partner Friend Other (specify): ______________

Instructions

You are being asked to describe the behavior of someone whom you know well. How often does that person experience each of these problems? Please circle the number next to each item that best describes their behavior **DURING THE PAST 6 MONTHS**. Please ignore the sections marked "Office Use Only."

	Section 1 Items	Never or rarely	Some-times	Often	Very often
1.	Procrastinates or puts off doing things until the last minute	1	2	3	4
2.	Poor sense of time	1	2	3	4
3.	Wastes or mismanages his/her time	1	2	3	4
4.	Not prepared on time for work or assigned tasks	1	2	3	4
5.	Fails to meet deadlines for assignments	1	2	3	4
6.	Has trouble planning ahead or preparing for upcoming events	1	2	3	4
7.	Forgets to do things he/she is supposed to do	1	2	3	4
8.	Can't seem to accomplish the goals he/she sets for self	1	2	3	4
9.	Late for work or scheduled appointments	1	2	3	4
10.	Can't seem to hold in mind things he/she needs to remember to do	1	2	3	4
11.	Can't seem to get things done unless there is an immediate deadline	1	2	3	4
12.	Has difficulty judging how much time it will take to do something or get somewhere	1	2	3	4
13.	Has trouble motivating self to start work	1	2	3	4
14.	Has difficulty motivating self to stick with his/her work and get it done	1	2	3	4
15.	Not motivated to prepare in advance for things he/she knows he/she is supposed to do	1	2	3	4
16.	Has trouble completing one activity before starting into a new one	1	2	3	4
17.	Has trouble doing what he/she tells self to do	1	2	3	4
18.	Difficulties following through on promises or commitments he/she may make to others	1	2	3	4
19.	Lacks self-discipline	1	2	3	4

(cont.)

20. Has difficulty arranging or doing his/her work by its priority or importance; can't "prioritize" well	1	2	3	4
21. Finds it hard to get started or get going on things he/she needs to get done	1	2	3	4
Office Use Only—**Section 1 Total Score** ________				
Section 2 Items	Never or rarely	Some-times	Often	Very often
22. Does not seem to anticipate the future as much or as well as others	1	2	3	4
23. Can't seem to remember what he/she previously heard or read about	1	2	3	4
24. Has trouble organizing his/her thoughts	1	2	3	4
25. When he/she is shown something complicated to do, he/she cannot keep the information in mind so as to imitate or do it correctly	1	2	3	4
26. Has trouble considering various options for doing things and weighing their consequences	1	2	3	4
27. Has difficulties saying what he/she wants to say	1	2	3	4
28. Unable to come up with or invent as many solutions to problems as others seem to do	1	2	3	4
29. Finds he/she is at a loss for words when he/she wants to explain something to others	1	2	3	4
30. Has trouble putting his/her thoughts down in writing as well or as quickly as others	1	2	3	4
31. Feels he/she is not as creative or inventive as others of his/her level of intelligence	1	2	3	4
32. In trying to accomplish goals or assignments, he/she finds that he/she is not able to think of as many ways of doing things as others	1	2	3	4
33. Has trouble learning new or complex activities as well as others	1	2	3	4
34. Has difficulty explaining things in their proper order or sequence	1	2	3	4
35. Can't seem to get to the point of his/her explanations as quickly as others	1	2	3	4
36. Has trouble doing things in their proper order or sequence	1	2	3	4
37. Unable to "think on his/her feet" or respond as effectively as others to unexpected events	1	2	3	4
38. Is slower than others at solving problems he/she encounters in his/her daily life	1	2	3	4
39. Easily distracted by irrelevant events or thoughts when he/she must concentrate on something	1	2	3	4
40. Not able to comprehend what he/she reads as well as he/she should be able to do; has to reread material to get its meaning	1	2	3	4

(cont.)

41. Cannot focus his/her attention on tasks or work as well as others	1	2	3	4
42. Easily confused	1	2	3	4
43. Can't seem to sustain his/her concentration on reading, paperwork, lectures, or work	1	2	3	4
44. Finds it hard to focus on what is important from what is not important when he/she does things	1	2	3	4
45. Doesn't seem to process information as quickly or as accurately as others	1	2	3	4
Office Use Only—**Section 2 Total Score** ______				
Section 3 Items	Never or rarely	Some-times	Often	Very often
46. Finds it difficult to tolerate waiting; impatient	1	2	3	4
47. Makes decisions impulsively	1	2	3	4
48. Unable to inhibit his/her reactions or responses to events or others	1	2	3	4
49. Has difficulty stopping his/her activities or behavior when he/she should do so	1	2	3	4
50. Has difficulty changing his/her behavior when he/she is given feedback about mistakes	1	2	3	4
51. Makes impulsive comments to others	1	2	3	4
52. Likely to do things without considering the consequences for doing them	1	2	3	4
53. Changes his/her plans at the last minute on a whim or last minute impulse	1	2	3	4
54. Fails to consider past relevant events or past personal experiences before responding to situations (Acts without thinking)	1	2	3	4
55. Not aware of things he/she says or does	1	2	3	4
56. Has difficulty being objective about things that affect him/her	1	2	3	4
57. Finds it hard to take other people's perspectives about a problem or situation	1	2	3	4
58. Doesn't think about or talk things over with self before doing something	1	2	3	4
59. Trouble following the rules in a situation	1	2	3	4
60. More likely to drive a motor vehicle much faster than others (Excessive speeding)	1	2	3	4
61. Has a low tolerance for frustrating situations	1	2	3	4
62. Cannot inhibit his/her emotions as well as others	1	2	3	4
63. Doesn't look ahead and think about what the future outcomes will be before he/she does something (Doesn't use his/her foresight)	1	2	3	4
64. Engages in risk taking activities more than others are likely to do	1	2	3	4

(cont.)

Office Use Only—**Section 3 Total Score** ________				
Section 4 Items	Never or rarely	Some-times	Often	Very often
65. Likely to take short cuts in his/her work and not do all that he/she is supposed to do	1	2	3	4
66. Likely to skip out on work early if his/her work is boring to do	1	2	3	4
67. Does not put as much effort into his/her work as he/she should or than others are able to do	1	2	3	4
68. Others tell him/her that he/she is lazy or unmotivated	1	2	3	4
69. Has to depend on others to help them get their work done	1	2	3	4
70. Things must have an immediate payoff for him/her or he/she does not seem to get them done	1	2	3	4
71. Has difficulty resisting the urge to do something fun or more interesting when he/she is supposed to be working	1	2	3	4
72. Inconsistent in the quality or quantity of his/her work performance	1	2	3	4
73. Unable to work as well as others without supervision or frequent instruction	1	2	3	4
74. Does not have the willpower or determination that others seem to have	1	2	3	4
75. Is not able to work toward longer term or delayed rewards as well as others	1	2	3	4
76. Cannot resist doing things that produce immediate rewards, even if those things are not good for him/her in the long run	1	2	3	4
Office Use Only—**Section 4 Total Score** ________				
Section 5 Items	Never or rarely	Some-times	Often	Very often
77. Quick to get angry or become upset	1	2	3	4
78. Overreacts emotionally	1	2	3	4
79. Easily excitable	1	2	3	4
80. Unable to inhibit showing strong negative or positive emotions	1	2	3	4
81. Has trouble calming self down once he/she is emotionally upset	1	2	3	4
82. Cannot seem to regain emotional control and become more reasonable once he/she is emotional	1	2	3	4
83. Cannot seem to distract self away from whatever is upsetting him/her emotionally to help calm self down. Can't refocus his/her mind to a more positive framework.	1	2	3	4
84. Unable to manage his/her emotions in order to accomplish his/her goals successfully or get along well with others	1	2	3	4

(cont.)

85. Remains emotional or upset longer than others	1	2	3	4
86. Finds it difficult to walk away from emotionally upsetting encounters with others or leave situations in which he/she has become very emotional	1	2	3	4
87. Cannot rechannel or redirect his/her emotions into more positive ways or outlets when he/she gets upset	1	2	3	4
88. Is not able to evaluate an emotionally upsetting event more objectively	1	2	3	4
89. Cannot redefine negative events into more positive viewpoints when he/she feels strong emotions	1	2	3	4
Office Use Only—**Section 5 Total Score** ________				
Office Use Only **Total of Sections 1–5: Total EF Summary Score** ________				
Office Use Only **Count number of items answered 3 or 4** **EF Symptom Count** ________				
Office Use Only **Add Items 1, 6, 14, 16, 24, 49, 50, 55, 60, 65, and 69** **ADHD-EF Index Score** ________				

BDEFS-LF: Self-Report Score Sheet for Raw Scores (Ages 18–34, Males Only)

Name: ______________________ Age: _____ Sex: _______ Date: ________

Raw Score Ranges and Percentiles

%	Self-Management to Time	Self-Organization/ Problem Solving	Self-Restraint	Self-Motivation	Self-Regulation of Emotions	Total EF Summary Score	ADHD-EF Index	%
99+	74–84	78–96	62–76	33–48	49–52	258–356	33–44	99+
98	64–73	74–77	55–61	31–32	46–48	243–257	31–32	98
97	63	61–73	51–54	—	40–45	229–242	30	97
96	61–62	60	50	30	37–39	214–228	29	96
95	60	57–59	49	29	36	202–213	28	95
94	59	55–56	48	—	35	199–201	27	94
93	58	54	46–47	28	34	198	26	93
92	57	51–53	44–45	27	32–33	197	25	92
91	56	—	—	—	30–31	196	—	91
90	55	50	43	26	29	195	—	90
89	—	49	41–42	25	28	194	24	89
88	54	48	40	24	27	190–193	—	88
87	53	—	—	—	—	189	—	87
86	—	—	39	—	—	184–188	23	86
85	52	—	—	—	—	183	—	85
84	51	—	38	23	26	181–182	—	84
83	50	47	—	—	—	179–180	—	83
82	48–49	—	—	22	—	178	—	82
81	—	—	—	—	—	176–177	22	81
80	47	46	—	—	—	173–175	—	80
79	—	—	—	—	25	171–172	—	79
78	46	45	—	21	—	169–170	—	78
77	45	—	—	—	—	167–168	21	77
76	44	44	37	—	24	165–166	—	76
51–75	34–43	33–43	29–36	15–20	17–23	134–164	18–20	51–75
26–50	28–33	27–32	23–28	13–14	14–16	109–133	14–17	26–50
1–25	21–27	24–26	19–22	12	13	89–108	11–13	1–25

BDEFS-LF: Self-Report Score Sheet for Raw Scores (Ages 18–34, Females Only)

Name: ______________________ Age: _____ Sex: ________ Date: ________

Raw Score Ranges and Percentiles

%	Self-Management to Time	Self-Organization/ Problem Solving	Self-Restraint	Self-Motivation	Self-Regulation of Emotions	Total EF Summary Score	ADHD-EF Index	%
99+	63–84	66–96	57–76	36–48	42–52	233–356	33–44	99+
98	61–62	63–65	53–56	34–35	40–41	231–232	31–32	98
97	58–60	62	51–52	32–33	39	223–230	30	97
96	57	59–61	48–50	29–31	37–38	211–222	29	96
95	56	58	47	27–28	36	207–210	28	95
94	—	56–57	45–46	25–26	34–35	206	27	94
93	55	54–55	43–44	24	33	199–205	26	93
92	53–54	53	41–42	—	—	195–198	25	92
91	—	52	—	—	32	192–194	—	91
90	—	51	40	23	31	188–191	—	90
89	52	50	39	22	—	186–187	24	89
88	—	—	—	—	30	184–185	—	88
87	51	—	38	21	—	180–183	—	87
86	50	—	—	—	—	179	23	86
85	49	48–49	—	20	29	178	—	85
84	—	—	—	19	—	—	—	84
83	48	—	—	—	—	175–177	—	83
82	47	47	—	—	—	174	—	82
81	45–46	—	—	—	28	173	22	81
80	—	—	37	18	—	172	—	80
79	44	46	—	—	—	171	—	79
78	43	—	—	—	—	—	—	78
77	—	45	—	17	—	170	21	77
76	—	—	36	—	26–27	167–169	—	76
51–75	36–42	36–44	27–35	15–16	20–25	132–166	18–20	51–75
26–50	28–35	27–35	23–26	13–14	15–19	111–131	14–17	26–50
1–25	21–27	24–26	19–22	12	13–14	89–110	11–13	1–25

BDEFS-LF: Self-Report Score Sheet for Raw Scores (Ages 18–34, Males and Females Combined)

Name: ______________________ Age: _____ Sex: _______ Date: ________

Raw Score Ranges and Percentiles

%	Self-Management to Time	Self-Organization/ Problem Solving	Self-Restraint	Self-Motivation	Self-Regulation of Emotions	Total EF Summary Score	ADHD-EF Index	%
99+	71–84	77–96	60–76	36–48	47–52	258–356	33–44	99+
98	63–70	67–76	57–59	32–35	42–46	233–257	31–32	98
97	61–62	63–66	53–56	31	40–41	229–232	30	97
96	60	60–62	50–52	29–30	38–39	214–228	29	96
95	58–59	58–59	49	—	36–37	207–213	28	95
94	57	56–57	47–48	28	35	202–206	27	94
93	56	54–55	45–46	27	34	198–201	26	93
92	—	52–53	44	26	33	—	25	92
91	55	51	43	25	32	196–197	—	91
90	54	—	42	24	31	194–195	—	90
89	53	50	41	—	30	190–193	24	89
88	—	—	39–40	—	—	188–189	—	88
87	52	49	—	—	29	185–187	—	87
86	—	48	—	23	—	182–184	23	86
85	51	—	38	22	28	180–181	—	85
84	50	—	—	—	—	179	—	84
83	48–49	47	—	21	—	178	—	83
82	—	—	—	—	27	176–177	—	82
81	47	—	—	20	—	174–175	22	81
80	46	—	—	—	26	172–173	—	80
79	45	46	—	—	—	171	—	79
78	—	45	37	19	—	170	—	78
77	44	—	—	—	—	169	21	77
76	43	—	—	—	—	167–168	—	76
51–75	35–42	35–44	28–36	15–18	18–25	133–166	18–20	51–75
26–50	28–34	27–34	23–27	13–14	15–17	110–132	14–17	26–50
1–25	21–27	24–26	19–22	12	13–14	89–109	11–13	1–25

BDEFS-LF: Self-Report Score Sheet for Raw Scores (Ages 35–49, Males Only)

Name: ______________________ Age: _____ Sex: _______ Date: ________

Raw Score Ranges and Percentiles

%	Self-Management to Time	Self-Organization/ Problem Solving	Self-Restraint	Self-Motivation	Self-Regulation of Emotions	Total EF Summary Score	ADHD-EF Index	%
99+	74–84	81–96	61–76	38–48	50–52	260–356	32–44	99+
98	72–73	72–80	56–60	34–37	41–49	252–259	31	98
97	64–71	71	54–55	33	39–40	—	29–30	97
96	62–63	61–70	53	31–32	37–38	244–251	28	96
95	61	58–60	49–52	30	34–36	225–243	27	95
94	57–60	55–57	48	28–29	33	214–224	26	94
93	55–56	53–54	43–47	25–27	32	198–213	25	93
92	52–54	51–52	42	24	—	193–197	24	92
91	49–51	—	41	—	31	188–192	—	91
90	48	—	—	23	—	185–187	23	90
89	—	50	40	22	—	183–184	22	89
88	47	49	39	21	30	179–182	21	88
87	46	48	—	—	—	177–178	—	87
86	45	46–47	38	20	—	175–176	—	86
85	44	—	—	—	—	173–174	—	85
84	—	45	—	19	29	170–172	—	84
83	—	44	37	—	—	167–169	20	83
82	—	—	—	—	28	165–166	—	82
81	43	43	36	18	27	164	—	81
80	—	—	—	—	26	163	—	80
79	42	42	35	—	—	161–162	19	79
78	—	—	34	—	25	159–160	—	78
77	41	—	—	17	—	157–158	—	77
76	—	—	33	—	—	155–156	—	76
51–75	32–40	30–41	26–32	14–16	16–24	117–154	16–18	51–75
26–50	25–31	25–29	21–25	13	14–15	100–116	13–15	26–50
1–25	21–24	24	19–20	12	13	89–99	11–12	1–25

BDEFS-LF: Self-Report Score Sheet for Raw Scores (Ages 35–49, Females Only)

Name: ______________________ Age: _____ Sex: _______ Date: _________

Raw Score Ranges and Percentiles

%	Self-Management to Time	Self-Organization/ Problem Solving	Self-Restraint	Self-Motivation	Self-Regulation of Emotions	Total EF Summary Score	ADHD-EF Index	%
99+	66–84	81–96	52–76	33–48	50–52	245–356	32–44	99+
98	62–65	69–80	50–51	30–32	45–49	232–244	31	98
97	61	62–68	46–49	29	41–44	230–231	29–30	97
96	57–60	60–61	45	24–28	37–40	220–229	28	96
95	56	59	44	23	35–36	214–219	27	95
94	54–55	55–58	41–43	22	34	206–213	26	94
93	51–53	—	39–40	19–21	32–33	197–205	25	93
92	—	51–54	—	—	30–31	179–196	24	92
91	50	48–50	38	—	—	171–178	—	91
90	45–49	—	37	—	29	169–170	23	90
89	44	—	—	—	—	168	22	89
88	—	47	—	18	—	167	21	88
87	—	45–46	36	17	28	163–166	—	87
86	43	43–44	35	—	—	160–162	—	86
85	—	—	—	—	27	157–159	—	85
84	—	42	—	—	26	156	—	84
83	42	—	—	—	—	155	20	83
82	41	—	34	16	25	154	—	82
81	40	41	—	—	—	152–153	—	81
80	—	—	—	—	—	149–151	—	80
79	39	40	33	—	—	146–148	19	79
78	—	—	32	—	24	—	—	78
77	—	—	—	—	—	145	—	77
76	—	—	31	—	—	142–144	—	76
51–75	32–38	33–39	27–30	14–15	18–23	125–141	16–18	51–75
26–50	26–31	27–32	21–26	13	14–17	104–124	13–15	26–50
1–25	21–25	24–26	19–20	12	13	89–103	11–12	1–25

BDEFS-LF: Self-Report Score Sheet for Raw Scores (Ages 35–49, Males and Females Combined)

Name: ______________________ Age: _____ Sex: _______ Date: ________

Raw Score Ranges and Percentiles

%	Self-Management to Time	Self-Organization/ Problem Solving	Self-Restraint	Self-Motivation	Self-Regulation of Emotions	Total EF Summary Score	ADHD-EF Index	%
99+	73–84	81–96	57–76	34–48	50–52	254–356	32–44	99+
98	65–72	73–80	54–56	33	41–49	244–253	31	98
97	62–64	69–72	51–53	31–32	40	233–243	29–30	97
96	61	61–68	49–50	30	37–39	223–232	28	96
95	58–60	59–60	46–48	29	34–36	216–222	27	95
94	55–57	56–58	43–45	24–28	33	210–215	26	94
93	53–54	54–55	41–42	—	32	198–209	25	93
92	51–52	51–53	—	23	—	193–197	24	92
91	50	—	39–40	22	31	185–192	—	91
90	48–49	50	—	21	30	180–184	23	90
89	47	48–49	38	20	—	176–179	22	89
88	45–46	—	—	19	—	172–175	21	88
87	44	46–47	—	—	29	170–171	—	87
86	—	—	37	—	—	168–169	—	86
85	—	45	—	18	28	166–167	—	85
84	43	44	36	—	—	164–165	—	84
83	—	43	—	—	27	161–163	20	83
82	—	42	35	17	26	159–160	—	82
81	42	—	—	—	—	158	—	81
80	41	—	34	—	25	155–157	—	80
79	—	—	—	—	—	—	19	79
78	40	41	33	—	—	153–154	—	78
77	—	—	—	16	—	152	—	77
76	39	40	32	—	24	150–151	—	76
51–75	32-38	32-39	26–31	14–15	17-23	121–149	16–18	51–75
26–50	25–31	26–31	21–25	13	14–16	102–120	13–15	26–50
1–25	21–24	24–25	19–20	12	13	89–101	11–12	1–25

BDEFS-LF: Self-Report Score Sheet for Raw Scores (Ages 50–64, Males Only)

Name: ______________________ Age: _____ Sex: ________ Date: _________

Raw Score Ranges and Percentiles

%	Self-Management to Time	Self-Organization/ Problem Solving	Self-Restraint	Self-Motivation	Self-Regulation of Emotions	Total EF Summary Score	ADHD-EF Index	%
99+	62–84	70–96	51–76	33–48	38–52	237–356	30–44	99+
98	59–61	69	49–50	29–32	36–37	226–236	28–29	98
97	57–58	66–68	46–48	28	35	214–225	27	97
96	56	63–65	45	—	—	212–213	26	96
95	55	62	44	27	33	200–211	—	95
94	54	59–61	—	26	31–32	195–199	25	94
93	52–53	56–58	43	24–25	30	191–194	24	93
92	51	—	—	23	29	—	—	92
91	—	55	42	—	27–28	186–190	23	91
90	50	53–54	40–41	22	—	181–185	—	90
89	48–49	52	—	—	26	180	22	89
88	46–47	50–51	—	—	—	179	—	88
87	—	48–49	39	21	—	176–178	—	87
86	—	—	—	20	25	171–175	21	86
85	45	46–47	38	—	—	165–170	—	85
84	—	—	—	—	24	163–164	—	84
83	44	45	—	19	—	161–162	—	83
82	43	44	—	—	—	160	—	82
81	42	—	36–37	18	—	159	—	81
80	41	—	35	—	—	158	—	80
79	40	43	—	—	23	157	20	79
78	—	—	—	—	22	155–156	—	78
77	—	42	34	17	—	154	—	77
76	—	—	—	—	—	150–153	—	76
51–75	33–39	33–41	27–33	15–16	17–21	126–149	16–19	51–75
26–50	27–32	27–32	23–26	13–14	14–16	106–125	13–15	26–50
1–25	21–26	24–26	19–22	12	13	89–105	11–12	1–25

BDEFS-LF: Self-Report Score Sheet for Raw Scores (Ages 50–64, Females Only)

Name: ______________________ Age: _____ Sex: _______ Date: ________

Raw Score Ranges and Percentiles

%	Self-Management to Time	Self-Organization/ Problem Solving	Self-Restraint	Self-Motivation	Self-Regulation of Emotions	Total EF Summary Score	ADHD-EF Index	%
99+	67–84	72–96	47–76	28–48	38–52	216–356	30–44	99+
98	62–66	71	44–46	25–27	35–37	214–215	28–29	98
97	61	69–70	42–43	—	—	213	27	97
96	59–60	66–68	41	24	34	210—212	26	96
95	53–58	65	40	23	32–33	205–209	—	95
94	52	63–64	—	22	31	204	25	94
93	51	59–62	39	21	29–30	202–203	24	93
92	50	53–58	38	—	28	193–201	—	92
91	49	52	—	—	—	184–192	23	91
90	—	—	37	20	27	176–183	—	90
89	—	51	—	—	—	—	22	89
88	48	50	—	19	—	174–175	—	88
87	47	49	36	—	26	172–173	—	87
86	46	—	—	—	—	169–171	21	86
85	45	48	—	—	—	167–168	—	85
84	42–44	—	35	18	25	165–166	—	84
83	—	—	—	—	—	164	—	83
82	—	—	—	17	—	162–163	—	82
81	—	—	34	—	—	161	—	81
80	—	—	—	—	—	160	—	80
79	—	47	—	—	—	—	20	79
78	—	—	—	—	—	—	—	78
77	—	46	—	16	24	157–159	—	77
76	—	45	—	—	—	156	—	76
51–75	33–41	34–44	27–33	14–15	18–23	128–155	16–19	51–75
26–50	26–32	28–33	23–26	13	15–17	109–127	13–15	26–50
1–25	21–25	24–27	19–22	12	13–14	89–108	11–12	1–25

BDEFS-LF: Self-Report Score Sheet for Raw Scores (Ages 50–64, Males and Females Combined)

Name: ______________________ Age: _____ Sex: ________ Date: ________

Raw Score Ranges and Percentiles

%	Self-Management to Time	Self-Organization/ Problem Solving	Self-Restraint	Self-Motivation	Self-Regulation of Emotions	Total EF Summary Score	ADHD-EF Index	%
99+	66–84	72–96	51–76	32–48	38–52	237–356	30–44	99+
98	61–65	70–71	46–50	28–31	36–37	216–236	28–29	98
97	58–60	67–69	45	27	34–35	213–215	27	97
96	56–57	65–66	44	25–26	—	210–212	26	96
95	54–55	63–64	43	—	33	205–209	—	95
94	53	60–62	42	24	32	203–204	25	94
93	51–52	58–59	41	23	30–31	195–202	24	93
92	—	56–57	40	22	29	191–194	—	92
91	50	53–55	—	—	28	185–190	23	91
90	49	52	39	21	27	181–184	—	90
89	—	51	—	—	26	178–180	22	89
88	48	50	38	20	—	176–177	—	88
87	46–47	49	—	—	—	174–175	—	87
86	—	—	37	—	—	171–173	21	86
85	45	48	—	19	25	167–170	—	85
84	—	—	36	—	—	165–166	—	84
83	43–44	—	—	18	—	163–164	—	83
82	42	47	35	—	—	161–162	—	82
81	—	46	—	-	24	160	—	81
80	—	45	—	17	—	—	—	80
79	—	44	34	—	—	159	20	79
78	—	—	—	—	—	157–158	—	78
77	41	43	—	—	23	156	—	77
76	—	—	—	—	—	155	—	76
51–75	33–40	34–42	27–33	14–16	18–22	127–154	16–19	51–75
26–50	26–32	28–33	23–26	13	15–17	107–126	13–15	26–50
1–25	21–25	24–27	19–22	12	13–14	89–106	11–12	1–25

BDEFS-LF: Self-Report Score Sheet for Raw Scores (Ages 65–81, Males Only)

Name: ______________________ Age: _____ Sex: ________ Date: ________

Raw Score Ranges and Percentiles

%	Self-Management to Time	Self-Organization/ Problem Solving	Self-Restraint	Self-Motivation	Self-Regulation of Emotions	Total EF Summary Score	ADHD-EF Index	%
99+	58–84	62–96	43–76	24–48	34–52	189–356	25–44	99+
98	55–57	58–61	42	23	32–33	186–188	—	98
97	50–54	56–57	41	22	31	183–185	23–24	97
96	48–49	54–55	—	—	30	182	—	96
95	47	53	40	—	29	178–181	22	95
94	46	52	39	21	28	176–177	—	94
93	—	—	38	20	27	173–175	21	93
92	45	51	37	—	26	171–172	—	92
91	44	—	—	—	—	169–170	—	91
90	43	50	—	—	—	168	—	90
89	—	49	36	19	—	166–167	20	89
88	—	48	—	—	—	165	—	88
87	42	—	35	—	25	163–164	—	87
86	41	—	—	—	—	—	19	86
85	—	47	—	18	24	162	—	85
84	40	46	34	—	—	161	—	84
83	—	—	—	—	—	160	—	83
82	—	45	—	17	23	—	—	82
81	—	44	33	—	—	159	—	81
80	—	—	—	—	22	158	—	80
79	—	43	—	—	—	155–157	—	79
78	39	—	—	—	—	154	18	78
77	—	—	—	—	21	153	—	77
76	—	—	—	—	—	151–152	—	76
51–75	31–38	34–42	28–32	14–16	17–20	125–150	16–17	51–75
26–50	26–30	28–33	23–27	13	14–16	105–124	13–15	26–50
1–25	21–25	24–27	19–22	12	13	89–104	11–12	1–25

BDEFS-LF: Self-Report Score Sheet for Raw Scores (Ages 65–81, Females Only)

Name: ______________________ Age: _____ Sex: _______ Date: ________

Raw Score Ranges and Percentiles

%	Self-Management to Time	Self-Organization/ Problem Solving	Self-Restraint	Self-Motivation	Self-Regulation of Emotions	Total EF Summary Score	ADHD-EF Index	%
99+	50–84	60–96	47–76	22–48	33–52	195–356	25–44	99+
98	48–49	58–59	45–46	21	30–32	186–194	—	98
97	47	57	43–44	20	28–29	178–185	23–24	97
96	46	56	41–42	—	27	174–177	—	96
95	—	55	38–40	—	—	171–173	22	95
94	45	54	37	—	—	167–170	—	94
93	—	53	—	—	—	165–166	21	93
92	44	50–52	—	19	26	163–164	—	92
91	43	—	36	—	—	162	—	91
90	—	49	—	—	25	160–161	—	90
89	42	47–48	35	18	—	158–159	20	89
88	41	—	34	—	—	157	—	88
87	—	—	—	—	24	156	—	87
86	—	—	33	—	—	154–155	19	86
85	40	—	—	—	—	153	—	85
84	—	46	—	17	23	152	—	84
83	39	—	32	—	—	151	—	83
82	38	—	—	16	22	—	—	82
81	37	45	—	—	—	149–150	—	81
80	—	—	31	—	—	147–148	—	80
79	—	—	—	—	—	—	—	79
78	36	44	—	—	21	146	18	78
77	—	43	30	15	—	145	—	77
76	35	42	—	—	—	144	—	76
51–75	31–34	36–41	26–29	14	17–20	123–143	16–17	51–75
26–50	27–30	30–35	22–25	13	14–16	109–122	13–15	26–50
1–25	21–26	24–29	19–21	12	13	89–108	11–12	1–25

BDEFS-LF: Self-Report Score Sheet for Raw Scores (Ages 65–81, Males and Females Combined)

Name: ______________________ Age: _____ Sex: ________ Date: ________

Raw Score Ranges and Percentiles

%	Self-Management to Time	Self-Organization/ Problem Solving	Self-Restraint	Self-Motivation	Self-Regulation of Emotions	Total EF Summary Score	ADHD-EF Index	%
99+	57–84	62–96	46–76	24–48	37–52	194–356	25–44	99+
98	51–56	58–61	43–45	22–23	32–36	186–193	—	98
97	48–50	57	42	—	30–31	183–185	23–24	97
96	47	56	41	21	29	178–182	—	96
95	46	55	40	20	28	176–177	22	95
94	—	53–54	39	—	27	172–175	—	94
93	45	52	37–38	—	—	170–171	21	93
92	—	51	—	—	26	168–169	—	92
91	44	50	—	—	—	166–167	—	91
90	43	—	36	19	—	165	—	90
89	—	48–49	—	—	25	163–164	20	89
88	42	—	35	—	—	162	—	88
87	41	47	—	18	—	161	—	87
86	—	—	34	—	24	160	19	86
85	—	—	—	—	—	159	—	85
84	40	46	33	—	—	158	—	84
83	—	—	—	17	23	156–157	—	83
82	—	45	—	—	—	154–155	—	82
81	—	—	—	—	22	153	—	81
80	39	44	—	—	—	151–152	—	80
79	—	—	—	—	—	—	—	79
78	38	43	32	16	—	150	18	78
77	—	—	—	—	21	148–149	—	77
76	37	42	—	—	—	146–147	—	76
51–75	31–36	35–41	27–31	14–15	17–20	124–145	16–17	51–75
26–50	27–30	29–34	23–26	13	14–16	108–123	13–15	26–50
1–25	21–26	24–28	19–22	12	13	89–107	11–12	1–25

BDEFS-LF: Self-Report Score Sheet for Total EF Symptom Counts (All Ages and Both Sexes)

Name: ______________________ Age: _____ Sex: _______ Date: _________

Total EF Symptom Counts and Percentiles

%	Ages 18–34	Ages 35–49	Ages 50–64	Ages 65–81	%
99+	63+	57+	51+	29+	99+
98	58–62	50–56	42–50	26–28	98
97	45–57	45–49	41	23–25	97
96	42–44	44	38–40	21–22	96
95	39–41	36–43	35–37	—	95
94	37–38	32–35	31–34	18–20	94
93	35–36	30–31	30	16–17	93
92	32–34	29	28–29	—	92
91	31	25–28	22–27	15	91
90	30	23–24	21	14	90
89	29	21–22	20	—	89
88	28	19–20	—	12–13	88
87	26–27	18	18–19	—	87
86	23–25	17	17	11	86
85	22	14–16	16	—	85
84	—	—	15	10	84
83	21	13	14	—	83
82	18–20	12	—	—	82
81	—	11	12–13	9	81
80	—	—	11	—	80
79	17	10	—	8	79
78	16	—	10	—	78
77	—	—	—	7	77
76	15	9	9	—	76
51–75	5–14	2–8	2–8	1–6	51–75
≤ 50	0–4	0–1	0–1	0	≤ 50

Note. A symptom is any item on the BDEFS answered with a 3 (often) or a 4 (very often).

BDEFS-SF: Self-Report

Name: ______________________ Date: ______________

Sex: (Circle one) Male Female Age: __________

Instructions

How often do you experience each of these problems? Please circle the number next to each item that best describes your behavior **DURING THE PAST 6 MONTHS**. Please ignore the sections marked "Office Use Only."

Short Form Items	Never or rarely	Some-times	Often	Very often
1. Procrastinate or put off doing things until the last minute	1	2	3	4
2. Can't seem to hold in mind things I need to remember to do	1	2	3	4
3. Not motivated to prepare in advance for things I know I am supposed to do	1	2	3	4
4. Have trouble doing what I tell myself to do	1	2	3	4
5. Have trouble learning new or complex activities as well as others	1	2	3	4
6. Have difficulty explaining things in their proper order or sequence	1	2	3	4
7. Unable to "think on my feet" or respond as effectively as others to unexpected events	1	2	3	4
8. I don't seem to process information as quickly or as accurately as others	1	2	3	4
9. Unable to inhibit my reactions or responses to events or others	1	2	3	4
10. Make impulsive comments to others	1	2	3	4
11. Likely to do things without considering the consequences for doing them	1	2	3	4
12. Fail to consider past relevant events or past personal experiences before responding to situations (I act without thinking)	1	2	3	4
13. Do not put as much effort into my work as I should or than others are able to do	1	2	3	4

(cont.)

14. Others tell me I am lazy or unmotivated	1	2	3	4
15. Inconsistent in the quality or quantity of my work performance	1	2	3	4
16. Unable to work as well as others without supervision or frequent instruction	1	2	3	4
17. Have trouble calming myself down once I am emotionally upset	1	2	3	4
18. Cannot seem to regain emotional control and become more reasonable once I am emotional	1	2	3	4
19. Cannot seem to distract myself away from whatever is upsetting me emotionally to help calm me down. I can't refocus my mind to a more positive framework.	1	2	3	4
20. I remain emotional or upset longer than others	1	2	3	4
Office Use Only—**Short Form Scores** Items 1–4 Score __________ Items 5–8 Score __________ Items 9–12 Score __________ Items 13–16 Score __________ Items 17–20 Score __________ Total EF Summary Score __________ EF Symptom Count __________				

BDEFS-SF: Other-Report

Name of person to be rated: ______________________ Date: ______________

Your name: ______________________________________

Your relationship to person being rated: (Circle one)

Mother Father Brother/sister Spouse/partner Friend Other (specify): ______________

Instructions

You are being asked to describe the behavior of someone whom you know well. How often does that person experience each of these problems? Please circle the number next to each item that best describes the person's behavior **DURING THE PAST 6 MONTHS**. Please ignore the sections marked "Office Use Only."

Short Form Items	Never or rarely	Some-times	Often	Very often
1. Procrastinates or puts off doing things until the last minute	1	2	3	4
2. Can't seem to hold in mind things he/she needs to remember to do	1	2	3	4
3. Not motivated to prepare in advance for things he/she knows he/she is supposed to do	1	2	3	4
4. Has trouble doing what he/she tells self to do	1	2	3	4
5. Has trouble learning new or complex activities as well as others	1	2	3	4
6. Has difficulty explaining things in their proper order or sequence	1	2	3	4
7. Unable to "think on his/her feet" or respond as effectively as others to unexpected events	1	2	3	4
8. Doesn't seem to process information as quickly or as accurately as others	1	2	3	4
9. Unable to inhibit his/her reactions or responses to events or others	1	2	3	4
10. Makes impulsive comments to others	1	2	3	4
11. Likely to do things without considering the consequences for doing them	1	2	3	4
12. Fails to consider past relevant events or past personal experiences before responding to situations (Acts without thinking)	1	2	3	4

(cont.)

13. Does not put as much effort into his/her work as he/she should or as others are able to do	1	2	3	4
14. Others tell him/her that he/she is lazy or unmotivated	1	2	3	4
15. Inconsistent in the quality or quantity of his/her work performance	1	2	3	4
16. Unable to work as well as others without supervision or frequent instruction	1	2	3	4
17. Has trouble calming self down once he/she is emotionally upset	1	2	3	4
18. Cannot seem to regain emotional control and become more reasonable once he/she is emotional	1	2	3	4
19. Cannot seem to distract self away from whatever is upsetting him/her emotionally to help calm self down. Can't refocus his/her mind to a more positive framework.	1	2	3	4
20. Remains emotional or upset longer than others	1	2	3	4
Office Use Only—**Short Form Scores** Items 1–4 Score ________ Items 5–8 Score ________ Items 9–12 Score ________ Items 13–16 Score ________ Items 17–20 Score ________ Total EF Summary Score ________ EF Symptom Count ________				

BDEFS-SF: Self-Report Score Sheet for Total EF Summary Scores and EF Symptom Counts (All Ages and Both Sexes)

Name: ______________________ Age: _____ Sex: ________ Date: _________

Raw Scores and Percentiles

	Ages 18–34		Ages 35–49		Ages 50–64		Ages 65–81		
%	Total EF Summary Score	EF Symptom Count	Total EF Summary Score	EF Symptom Count	Total EF Summary Score	EF Symptom Count	Total EF Summary Score	EF Symptom Count	%
99+	58–80	14–20	58–80	14–20	56–80	13–20	45–80	9–20	99+
98	52–57	12–13	54–57	12–13	51–55	11–12	42–44	6–8	98
97	50–51	11	53	10–11	49–50	10	41	5	97
96	48–49	9–10	51–52	9	48	9	40	—	96
95	47	—	49–50	8	47	8	—	4	95
94	46	8	47–48	7	44–46	7	39	—	94
93	45	—	45–46	—	42–43	—	38	—	93
92	44	7	44	—	41	6	—	—	92
91	43	—	43	6	—	5	37	—	91
90	—	—	41–42	—	40	—	—	—	90
89	42	6	40	—	—	—	—	3	89
88	—	—	—	5	—	4	36	—	88
87	—	—	39	—	39	—	—	—	87
86	—	—	—	4	38	—	—	—	86
85	41	5	38	—	—	—	35	2	85
84	40	—	37	—	—	—	—	—	84
83	—	4	—	—	37	—	34	—	83
82	—	—	36	3	—	—	—	—	82
81	39	—	—	—	36	3	—	—	81
80	—	—	35	2	—	—	—	—	80
79	—	—	—	—	—	—	33	—	79
78	38	—	34	—	35	—	—	1	78
77	—	3	—	—	—	2	—	—	77
76	37	—	33	—	—	—	—	—	76
51–75	29–36	1–2	27–32	1	28–34	1	27–32	0	51–75
26–50	24–28	0	23–26	0	24–27	0	24–26	—	26–50
1–25	20–23	—	20–22	—	20–23	—	20–23	—	1–25

Note. A symptom is any item on the BDEFS answered with a 3 (often) or a 4 (very often).

BDEFS-SF: Clinical Interview: Self-Report

Name of person being interviewed: ______________________________

Person's sex: (Circle one) Male Female Person's age: __________

Name of interviewer: ______________________________ Date: ______________

Instructions to Interviewer

Say the following to the person to be interviewed: "I would like to ask you a number of questions about your behavior during the past 6 months. For each behavior I ask you about, I want to know if it occurs *often or more frequently*." Place a check mark (✓) in the box after each item indicating the answer of the person being interviewed. Each item is simply answered Yes or No.

Interview Questions	No, this does not occur often	Yes, this occurs often or very often
1. Do you often procrastinate or put off doing things until the last minute?		
2. Do you often find that you can't seem to hold in mind things you need to remember to do?		
3. Do you often find that you are not motivated to prepare in advance for things you know you are supposed to do?		
4. Do you often have trouble doing what you tell yourself to do?		
5. Do you often have trouble learning new or complex activities as well as others?		
6. Do you often have difficulty explaining things in their proper order or sequence?		
7. Do you often find that you are unable to "think on your feet" or respond as effectively as others to unexpected events?		
8. Do you often find that you don't seem to process information as quickly or as accurately as others?		
9. Are you often unable to inhibit your reactions or responses to events or others?		
10. Do you often make impulsive comments to others?		
11. Are you often likely to do things without considering the consequences for doing them?		
12. Do you often fail to consider past relevant events or past personal experiences before responding to situations? In other words, do you often act without thinking?		

(cont.)

Interview Questions	No, this does not occur often	Yes, this occurs often or very often
13. Do you often find that you do not put as much effort into your work as you should or than others are able to do?		
14. Do others often tell you that you are lazy or unmotivated?		
15. Are you often inconsistent in the quality or quantity of your work performance?		
16. Are you often unable to work as well as others without supervision or frequent instruction?		
17. Do you often have trouble calming yourself down once you are emotionally upset?		
18. Do you often find that you cannot seem to regain emotional control and become more reasonable once you are emotional?		
19. Do you often find that you cannot seem to distract yourself away from whatever is upsetting you emotionally to help calm yourself down? In other words, you often can't refocus your mind to a more positive framework?		
20. Do you often remain emotional or upset longer than others?		
Office Use Only—**Clinical Interview Score** EF Symptom Count ________		

References

Abidin, R. R. (1995). *The Parenting Stress Index—Short Form.* Odessa, FL: Psychological Assessment Resources.

Alderman, N., Burgess, P. W., Knight, C., & Henman, C. (2003). Ecological validity of a simplified version of the Multiple Errands Shopping Test. *Journal of the International Neuropsychological Society, 9,* 31–44.

American Educational Research Association, American Psychological Association, & National Council on Measurement in Education. (1999). *Standards for educational and psychological testing* (2nd ed.). Washington, DC: American Educational Research Association.

American Psychiatric Association. (2000). *Diagnostic and statistical manual of mental disorders* (4th ed.). Washington, DC: Author.

Anderson, P. (2002). Assessment and development of executive function (EF) during childhood. *Child Neuropsychology, 8,* 71–82.

Anderson, V. A., Anderson, P., Northam, E., Jacobs, R., & Mikiewicz, O. (2002). Relationships between cognitive and behavioral measures of executive function in children with brain disease. *Child Neuropsychology, 8,* 231–240.

Baddeley, A. D. (1986). *Working memory.* Oxford, UK: Clarendon Press.

Barkley, R. A. (1987). Child behavior rating scales and checklists. In M. Rutter, H. Tuma, & I. Lann (Eds.), *Assessment and diagnosis in child and adolescent psychopathology* (pp. 113–155). New York: Guilford Press.

Barkley, R. A. (1991). The ecological validity of laboratory and analogue assessments of ADHD symptoms. *Journal of Abnormal Child Psychology, 19,* 149–178.

Barkley, R. A. (1994). Impaired delayed responding: A unified theory of attention deficit hyperactivity disorder. In D. K. Routh (Ed.), *Disruptive behavior disorders in childhood: Essays honoring Herbert C. Quay* (pp. 11–57). New York: Plenum Press.

Barkley, R. A. (1997a). *ADHD and the nature of self-control.* New York: Guilford Press.

Barkley, R. A. (1997b). Inhibition, sustained attention, and executive functions: Constructing a unifying theory of ADHD. *Psychological Bulletin, 121,* 65–94.

Barkley, R. A. (2001). Executive functions and self-regulation: An evolutionary neuropsychological perspective. *Neuropsychology Review, 11,* 1–29.

Barkley, R.A. (2006). *Attention-deficit hyperactivity disorder: A handbook for diagnosis and treatment* (3rd ed.) New York: Guilford Press.

Barkley, R. A. (2010). Deficient emotional self-regulation: A core component of attention-deficit/hyperactivity disorder. *Journal of ADHD and Related Disorders, 1*(2), 5–37.

Barkley, R. A. (2011a). *Barkley Functional Impairment Scale (BFIS).* New York: Guilford Press.

Barkley, R. A. (2011b). *Executive functioning in everyday life.* New York: Guilford Press.

Barkley, R. A., & Cox, D. J. (2007). A review of driving risks and impairments associated with attention-deficit/hyperactivity disorder and the effects of stimulant medication on driving performance. *Journal of Safety Research, 38,* 113–128.

Barkley, R. A., & Fischer, M. (in press). Predicting impairment in occupational functioning in hyperactive children as adults: Self-reported executive function (EF) deficits vs. EF tests. *Developmental Neuropsychology.*

Barkley, R. A., Knouse, L. E., & Murphy, K. R. (in press). Correspondence and disparity in the self and other ratings of current and childhood symptoms and impairments in adults with ADHD. *Psychological Assessment.*

Barkley, R. A., & Murphy, K. R. (2006). *Attention-deficit hyperactivity disorder: A clinical workbook* (3rd ed.). New York: Guilford Press.

Barkley, R. A., & Murphy, K. R. (2010a). Impairment in occupational functioning and adult ADHD: The predictive utility of executive function (EF) ratings versus EF tests. *Archives of Clinical Neuropsychology, 25*(3), 157–173.

Barkley, R. A., & Murphy, K. R. (2010b). *The nature of executive function (EF) deficits in daily life activities in adults with ADHD and their relationship to EF tests.* Manuscript submitted for publication.

Barkley, R. A., Murphy, K. R., DuPaul, G. I., & Bush, T. (2002). Driving in young adults with attention deficit hyperactivity disorder: Knowledge, performance, adverse outcomes, and the role of executive functioning. *Journal of the International Neuropsychological Society, 8,* 655–672.

Barkley, R. A., Murphy, K. R., & Fischer, M. (2008). *ADHD in adults: What the science says.* New York: Guilford Press.

Bekhterev, V. M. (1905–1907). *Fundamentals of brain function.* St. Petersburg, Russia: Brokhauz i Efron.

Bianchi, L. (1922). *The mechanism of the brain and the function of the frontal lobes.* Edinburgh, UK: Livingstone.

Biederman, J., Petty, C. R., Fried, R., Black, S., Faneuil, A., Doyle, A. E., et al. (2008). Discordance between psychometric testing and questionnaire-based definitions of executive function deficits in individuals with ADHD. *Journal of Attention Disorders, 12,* 92–102.

Biederman, J., Petty, C. R., Fried, R., Doyle, A. E., Mick, E., Aleardi, M., et al. (2008). Utility of an abbreviated questionnaire to identify individuals with ADHD at risk for functional impairments. *Journal of Psychiatric Research, 42*(4), 304–310.

Biederman, J., Petty, C., Fried, R., Fontanella, J., Doyle, A. E., Seidman, L. J., et al. (2006). Impact of psychometrically defined deficits of executive functioning in adults with attention deficit hyperactivity disorder. *American Journal of Psychiatry, 163,* 1730–1738.

Bogod, N. M., Mateer, C. A., & MacDonald, S. W. S. (2003). Self-awareness after traumatic brain injury: A comparison of measures and their relationship to executive functions. *Journal of the International Neuropsychological Society, 9,* 450–458.

Boonstra, A. M., Oosterlaan, J., Sergeant, J. A., & Buitelaar, J. K. (2005). Executive functioning in adult ADHD: A meta-analytic review. *Psychological Medicine, 35,* 1097–1108.

Borkowski, J. G., & Burke, J. E. (1996). Theories, models, and measurements of executive functioning: An information processing perspective. In G. R. Lyon & N. A. Krasnegor (Eds.), *Attention, memory, and executive functioning* (pp. 235–262). Baltimore: Brookes.

Bryant, F. B. (2000). Assessing the validity of measurement. In. L. G. Grim & P. R. Yarnold (Eds.), *Reading and understanding more multivariate statistics* (pp. 99–146). Washington, DC: American Psychological Association.

Buckholtz, J. W., Treadway, M. T., Cowan, R. L., Woodward, N. D., Li, R., Ansari, M. S., et al. (2010). Dopaminergic network differences in human impulsivity. *Science, 319,* 532.

Burgess, P. W., Alderman, N., Evans, J., Emslie, H., & Wilson, B. A. (1998). The ecological validity of tests of executive function. *Journal of the International Neuropsychological Society, 4,* 547–558.

Bush, G., Valera, E. M., & Seidman, L. J. (2005). Functional neuroimaging of attention-deficit/hyperactivity disorder: A review and suggested future directions. *Biological Psychiatry, 57,* 1273–1296.

Butterfield, E. C., & Albertson, L. R. (1995). On making cognitive theory more general and developmentally pertinent. In F. Weinert & W. Schneider (Eds.), *Research on memory development* (pp. 73–99). Hillsdale, NJ: Erlbaum.

Butterfield, E. C., & Belmont, J. M. (1977). Assessing and improving the executive cognitive functions of mentally retarded persons. In I. Bialer & M. Steinlich (Eds.), *The psychology of mental retardation* (pp. 277–307). New York: Psychological Dimensions.

Cairns, R. B., & Green, J. A. (1979). How to assess personality and social patterns: Observations or ratings? In R. B. Cairns (Ed.), *The analysis of social interactions* (pp. 209–226). Hillsdale, NJ: Erlbaum.

Castellanos, X., Sonuga-Barke, E., Milham, M., & Tannock, R. (2006). Characterizing cognition in ADHD: Beyond executive dysfunction. *Trends in Cognitive Sciences, 10,* 117–123.

Chaytor, N., Schmitter-Edgecombe, M., & Burr, R. (2006). Improving the ecological validity of executive functioning assessment. *Archives of Clinical Neuropsychology, 21,* 217–227.

Ciairano, S., Visu-Petra, L., & Settanni, M. (2007). Executive inhibitory control and cooperative behavior during early school years: A follow-up study. *Journal of Abnormal Child Psychology, 35,* 335–345.

Conners, C. K. (1995). *The Conners Continuous Performance Test.* North Tonawanda, NY: Multi-Health Systems.

Cook, T. D., & Campbell, D. T. (1979). *Quasi-experimentation: Design and analysis issues for field settings.* Chicago: Rand McNally.

Denckla, M. B. (1996). A theory and model of executive function: A neuropsychological perspective. In G. R. Lyon & N. A. Krasnegor (Eds.), *Attention, memory, and executive function* (pp. 263–278). Baltimore: Brookes.

Derogatis, L. (1986). *Manual for the Symptom Checklist 90—Revised (SCL-90-R).* Baltimore: Author.

Dimond, S. J. (1980). *Neuropsychology: A textbook of systems and psychological functions of the human brain.* London: Butterworths.

Dodrill, C. B. (1997). Myths of neuropsychology. *The Clinical Neuropsychologist, 11,* 1–17.

Eslinger, P. J. (1996). Conceptualizing, describing, and measuring components of executive function: A summary. In G. R. Lyon & N. A. Krasnegor (Eds.), *Attention, memory, and executive function* (pp. 367–395). Baltimore: Brookes.

Frazier, T. W., Demareem, H. A., & Youngstrom, E. A. (2004). Meta-analysis of intellectual and neuropsychological test performance in attention-deficit/hyperactivity disorder. *Neuropsychology, 18,* 543–555.

Friedman, H. S., Tucker, J. S., Schwartz, J. E., Tomlinson-Keasey, C., Martin, L. R., Wingard, D. L., et al. (1995). Psychosocial and behavioral predictors of longevity: The aging and death of the "Termites." *American Psychologist, 50,* 69–78.

Fuster, J. (1980). *The prefrontal cortex.* New York: Raven Press.

Fuster, J. M. (1997). *The prefrontal cortex* (3rd ed.). Philadelphia: Lippincott-Raven.

Gilotty, L., Kenworthy, L., Sirian, L., Black, D. O., & Wagner, A. E. (2002). Adaptive skills and executive function in autism spectrum disorders. *Child Neuropsychology, 8,* 241–248.

Gioia, G. A., Isquith, P. K., Guy, S. C., & Kenworthy, L. (2000). *BRIEF: Behavior Rating Inventory of Executive Function—Professional Manual.* Odessa, FL: Psychological Assessment Resources.

Gioia, G. A., Isquith, P. K., Kenworthy, L., & Barton, R. M. (2002). Profiles of everyday executive function in acquired and developmental disorders. *Child Neuropsychology, 8,* 121–137.

Gottman, J., & Katz, L. (1989). Effects of marital discord on young children's peer interaction and health. *Developmental Psychology, 25,* 373–381.

Green, L., Fry, A. F., & Myerson, J. (1994). Discounting of delayed rewards: A life-span comparison. *Psychological Science, 5,* 33–36.

Green, L., Myerson, J., Lichtman, D., Rosen, S., & Fry, A. (1996). Temporal discounting in choice delayed rewards: The role of age and income. *Psychology and Aging, 11,* 79–84.

Gropper, R. J., & Tannock, R. (2009). A pilot study of working memory and academic achievement in college students with ADHD. *Journal of Attention Disorders, 12,* 574–581.

Gross, J. J. (1998). The emerging field of emotion regulation: An integrative review. *Review of General Psychology, 2,* 271–299.

Gross, J. J., & John, O. P. (2003). Individual differences in two emotion regulation processes: Implications for affect, relationships, and well-being. *Journal of Personality and Social Psychology, 85,* 348–362.

Gross, J. J., & Thompson, R. A. (2007). Emotion regulation: Conceptual foundations. In J. J. Gross (Ed.), *Handbook of emotion regulation* (pp. 3–24). New York: Guilford Press.

Harlow, J. M. (1848). Passage of an iron rod through the head. *Boston Medical and Surgical Journal, 39,* 389–393.

Harlow, J. M. (1868). Recovery from the passage of an iron rod through the head. *Publications of the Massachusetts Medical Society, 2,* 237–346.

Hayes, S. C. (1989). *Rule-governed behavior: Cognition, contingencies, and instructional control.* New York: Plenum Press.

Hayes, S. C., Gifford, E. V., & Ruckstuhl, L. E., Jr. (1996). Relational frame theory and executive functioning: A behavioral approach. In G. R. Lyon & N. A. Krasnegor (Eds.), *Attention, memory, and executive function* (pp. 279–305). Baltimore: Brookes.

Heaton, R. K. (1981). *A manual for the Wisconsin Card Sorting Test.* Odessa, FL: Psychological Assessment Resources.

Heilman, K. (1994, January). *Intention.* Paper presented at the NICHD Conference on Attention, Memory, and Executive Function, Bethesda, MD.

Hervey, A. S., Epstein, J. N., & Curry, J. F. (2004). Neuropsychology of adults with attention-deficit/hyperactivity disorder: A meta-analytic review. *Neuropsychology, 18,* 495–503.

Hinshaw, S. P. (2003). Impulsivity, emotion regulation, and developmental psychopathology: Specific versus generality of linkages. *Annals of the New York Academy of Sciences, 1008,* 149–159.

Hinshaw, S. P., Carte, E. T., Fan, C., Jassy, J. S., & Owen, E. B. (2007). Neuropsychological functioning of girls with attention-deficit/hyperactivity disorder followed prospectively into adolescence: Evidence for continuing deficits? *Neuropsychology, 21,* 263–273.

Hollingshead, J. (1975). *A four-factor index of social position.* Unpublished manuscript, Yale University.

Hutchinson, A. D., Mathias, J. L., & Banich, M. T. (2008). Corpus callosum morphology in children and adolescents with attention deficit hyperactivity disorder: A meta-analytic review. *Neuropsychology, 22,* 341–349.

Jacobson, N. S., Roberts, L. J., Berns, S. B., & McGlinchey, J. B. (1999). Methods for defining and determining the clinical significance of treatment effects: Description, application, and alternatives. *Journal of Consulting and Clinical Psychology, 67,* 300–307.

Jacobson, N. S., & Truax, P. (1991). Clinical significance: A statistical approach to defining meaningful change in psychotherapy research. *Journal of Consulting and Clinical Psychology, 59,* 12–19.

Jastak, J., & Wilkinson, G. (1993). *Wide Range Achievement Test 3.* Wilmington, DE: Jastak Associates.

Jonsdottir, S., Bouma, A., Sergeant, J. A., & Scherder, E. J. A. (2006). Relationship between neuropsychological measures of executive function and behavioral measures of ADHD symptoms and comorbid behavior. *Archives of Clinical Neuropsychology, 21,* 383–394.

Kaufman, A. S., & Kaufman, N. L. (1993). *Kaufman Brief Intelligence Test.* Circle Pines, MN: American Guidance Service.

Kertesz, A., Nadkarni, N., Davidson, W., & Thomas, A. W. (2000). The Frontal Lobe Inventory in the differential diagnosis of frontotemporal dementia. *Journal of the International Neuropsychological Society, 6,* 460–468.

Kessler, R. C., Adler, L., Barkley, R. A., Biederman, J., Conners, C. K., Demler, O., et al. (2006). The prevalence and correlates of adult ADHD in the United States: Results from the National Comorbidity Survey Replication. *American Journal of Psychiatry, 163,* 716–723.

Lee, G. P., Strauss, E., Loring, D. W., McCloskey, L., Haworth, J. M., & Lehman, R. A. W. (1997). Sensitivity of figural fluency on the Five-Points Test to focal neurological dysfunction. *The Clinical Neuropsychologist, 11,* 59–68.

Lezak, M. D. (1995). *Neuropsychological assessment* (3rd ed.). New York: Oxford University Press.

Lezak, M. D., Howieson, D. B., Loring, D. W., Hannay, H. J., & Fischer, J. S. (2004). *Neuropsychological assessment* (4th ed.). New York: Oxford University Press.

Locke, H. J., & Wallace, K. M. (1959). Short marital adjustment and prediction tests: Their reliability and validity. *Journal of Marriage and Family Living, 21,* 251–255.

Luria, A. R. (1966). *Higher cortical functions in man.* New York: Basic Books.

Lyon, G. R., & Krasnegor, N. A. (Eds.). (1996). *Attention, memory, and executive function.* Baltimore: Brookes.

Mackie, S., Shaw, P., Lenroot, R., Greenstein, D. K., Nugent, T. F., III, Sharp, W. S., et al. (2007). Cerebellar development and clinical outcome in attention deficit hyperactivity disorder. *American Journal of Psychiatry, 76,* 647–655.

Mahone, E. M., Hagelthora, K. M., Cutting, L. E., Schuerholz, L. J., Pelletier, S. F., Rawlins, C., et al. (2002). Effects of IQ on executive function measures in children with ADHD. *Child Neuropsychology, 8,* 52–65.

Mangeot, S., Armstrong, K., Colvin, A. N., Yeates, K. O., & Taylor, H. G. (2002). Long-term executive function deficits in children with traumatic brain injuries: Assessment using the Behavior Rating Inventory of Executive Function (BRIEF). *Child Neuropsychology, 8,* 271–284.

Martel, M. M. (2009). Research review. A new perspective on attention-deficit/hyperactivity disorder: Emotion dysregulation and trait models. *Journal of Child Psychology and Psychiatry, 50,* 1042–1051.

Martel, M. M., Nikolas, M., & Nigg, J. T. (2007). Executive functions in adolescents with ADHD. *Journal of the American Academy of Child and Adolescent Psychiatry, 46,* 1437–1444.

Masters, J. C. (1991). Strategies and mechanisms for the personal and social control of emotion. In J. Garber & K. A. Dodge (Eds.), *The development of emotion regulation and dysregulation.* New York: Cambridge University Press.

Melnick, S. M., & Hinshaw, S. P. (2000). Emotion regulation and parenting in AD/HD and comparison boys: Linkages with social behaviors and peer preference. *Journal of Abnormal Child Psychology, 28,* 73–86.

Mises, L. von. (1990). *Human action: A treatise on economics* (3rd ed.). San Francisco: Laissez-Faire Books. (Original work published 1948)

Mitchell, J. T., Knouse, L. E., Nelson-Gray, R. O., & Kwapil, T. R. (2009). Self-reported ADHD symptoms among college students: Item position affects symptom endorsement rates. *Journal of Attention Disorders, 13,* 154–160.

Mitchell, M., & Miller, S. (2008). Executive functioning and observed versus self-reported measures of functional ability. *The Clinical Neuropsychologist, 22,* 471–479.

Multi-Health Systems. (1995). *The Learning and Memory Battery.* North Tonawanda, NY: Author.

Murphy, K. R., & Barkley, R. A. (1996). Prevalence of DSM-IV ADHD symptoms in adult licensed drivers. *Journal of Attention Disorders, 1,* 147–161.

Murphy, K. R., Barkley, R. A., & Bush, T. (2001). Executive functioning and olfactory identification in young adults with attention deficit hyperactivity disorder. *Neuropsychology, 15,* 211–220.

Nigg, J. T. (2006). *What Causes ADHD?: Understanding what goes wrong and why.* New York: Guilford Press.

Nigg, J. T., & Casey, B. J. (2005). An integrative theory of attention-deficit/hyperactivity disorder based on the cognitive and affective neurosciences. *Development and Psychopathology, 17,* 765–806.

Nigg, J. T., Willcutt, E. G., Doyle, A. E., & Sonuga-Barke, J. S. (2005). Causal heterogeneity in attention-deficit/hyperactivity disorder: Do we need neuropsychologically impaired subtypes? *Biological Psychiatry, 57,* 1224–1230.

Norman, D. A., & Shallice, T. (1986). Attention to action: Willed and automatic control of behavior. In R. J. Davidson, G. E. Schwartz, & D. Shapiro (Eds.), *Consciousness and self-regulation: Advances in research and theory* (Vol. 4, pp. 1–18). New York: Plenum Press.

Paloyelis, Y., Mehta, M. A., Kuntsi, J., & Asherson, P. (2007). Functional MRI in ADHD: A systematic literature review. *Expert Reviews in Neurotherapeutics, 7,* 1337–1356.

Pennington, B. F. (1997). Dimensions of executive functions in normal and abnormal development. In G. R. Lyon & N. A. Krasnegor (Eds.), *Development of the prefrontal cortex: Evolution, neurobiology, and behavior* (pp. 265–281). Baltimore: Brookes.

Pennington, B. F., Bennetto, L., McAleer, O., & Roberts, R. F. (1996). Executive functions and working memory: Theoretical and measurement issues. In G. R. Lyon & N. Krasnegor (Eds.), *Attention, memory, and executive function* (pp. 327–348). Baltimore: Brookes.

Pennington, B. F., & Ozonoff, S. (1996). Executive functions and developmental psychopathology. *Journal of Child Psychology and Psychiatry, 37,* 51–87.

Piatt, A. L., Fields, J. A., Paolo, A. M., & Troster, A. I. (1999). Action (verb naming) fluency as an executive function measure: Convergent and divergent evidence of validity. *Neuropsychologia, 27,* 1499–1503.

Pontius, A. A. (1973). Dysfunction patterns analogous to frontal lobe system and caudate nucleus syndromes in some groups of minimal brain dysfunction. *Journal of the American Medical Women's Association, 26,* 285–292.

Popper, K. (1979). *Objective knowledge: An evolutionary approach* (rev. ed.). Oxford, UK: Clarendon Press.

Pribram, K. H. (1973). The primate frontal cortex: Executive of the brain. In K. H. Pribram

& A. R. Luria (Eds.), *Psychophysiology of the frontal lobes* (pp. 293–314). New York: Academic Press.

Pribram, K. H. (1976). Executive functions of the frontal lobes. In T. Desiraju (Ed.), *Mechanisms in transmission of signals for conscious behaviour.* Amsterdam: Elsevier.

Regard, M., Strauss, E., & Knapp, P. (1982). Children's production on verbal and non-verbal fluency tasks. *Perceptual and Motor Skills, 123,* 17–22.

Reynolds, C., & Kamphaus, R. (1992). *Behavior Assessment System for Children.* Circle Pines, MN: American Guidance Service.

Rhodes, S., Coghill, D. R., & Matthews, K. (2005). Neuropsychological functioning in stimulant-naïve boys with hyperkinetic disorder. *Psychological Medicine, 35,* 1109–1120.

Riccio, C. A., Hall, J., Morgan, A., Hynd, G. W., & Gonzalez, J. J. (1994). Executive function and the Wisconsin Card Sort Test: Relationship with behavioral ratings and cognitive ability. *Developmental Neuropsychology, 10,* 215–229.

Roberts, R. J., & Pennington, B. F. (1996). An integrative framework for examining prefrontal cognitive processes. *Developmental Neuropsychology, 12,* 105–126.

Roth, R. M., Isquith, P. K., & Gioia, G. A. (2005). *Behavior Rating Inventory of Executive Function—Adult Version.* Lutz, FL: Psychological Assessment Resources.

Ruff, R. M., Allen, C. C., Farrow, C. E., Nieman, H., & Wylie, T. (1994). Figural fluency: Differential impairment in patients with left versus right frontal lesions. *Archives of Clinical Neuropsychology, 9,* 41–55.

Sagvolden, T., Johansen, E. B., Aase, H., & Russell, V. A. (2005). A dynamic developmental theory of attention-deficit/hyperactivity disorder (ADHD) predominantly hyperactive/impulsive and combined subtypes. *Behavioral and Brain Sciences, 25,* 397–468.

Seidman, L. J., Biederman, J., Valera, E. M., Monuteaux, M. C., Doyle, A. E., & Faraone, S. V. (2006). Neuropsychological functioning in girls with attention-deficit/hyperactivity disorder with and without learning disabilities. *Neuropsychology, 20,* 166–177.

Shallice, T. (1994). Multiple levels of control processes. In C. Umilta & M. Moscovitch (Eds.), *Attention and performance XV* (pp. 395–420). Cambridge, MA: MIT Press.

Shallice, T., & Burgess, P. W. (1991). Deficits in strategy application following frontal lobe damage in man. *Brain, 114,* 727–741.

Shelton, T. L., Barkley, R. A., Crosswait, C., Moorehouse, M., Fletcher, K., Barrett, S., et al. (1998). Psychiatric and psychological morbidity as a function of adaptive disability in preschool children with high levels of aggressive and hyperactive–impulsive–inattentive behavior. *Journal of Abnormal Child Psychology, 26,* 475–494.

Skinner, B. F. (1953). *Science and human behavior.* New York: Macmillan.

Skinner, H. A. (1994). *Computerized Lifestyle Assessment.* North Tonawanda, NY: Multi-Health Systems.

Stavro, G. M., Ettenhofer, M. L., & Nigg, J. T. (2007). Executive functions and adaptive functioning in young adults with attention-deficit/hyperactivity disorder. *Journal of the International Neuropsychological Society, 13,* 324–334.

Stroop, J. P. (1935). Studies of interference in serial verbal reactions. *Journal of Experimental Psychology, 18,* 643–662.

Stuss, D. T., & Benson, D. F. (1986). *The frontal lobes.* New York: Raven Press.

Thorell, L. B. (2007). Do delay aversion and executive function deficits make distinct contributions to the functional impact of ADHD symptoms?: A study of early academic skill deficits. *Journal of Child Psychology and Psychiatry, 48,* 1061–1070.

Thorell, L. B., Eninger, L., Brocki, K. C., & Bohlin, G. (2010). Childhood Executive Function Inventory (CHEXI): A promising measure for identifying young children with ADHD? *Journal of Clinical and Experimental Neuropsychology, 32,* 38–43.

Trenerry, M., Crosson, B., Deboe, J., & Leber, W. (1989). *Stroop Neuropsychological Screening Test.* Odessa, FL: Psychological Assessment Resources.

Valera, E. M., Faraone, S. V., Murray, K. E., & Seidman, L. J. (2007). Meta-analysis of structural imaging findings in attention-deficit/hyperactivity disorder. *Biological Psychiatry, 61,* 1361–1369.

Vriezen, E. R., & Pigott, S. E. (2002). The relationship between parental report on the BRIEF and performance-based measures of executive function in children with moderate to severe traumatic brain injury. *Child Neuropsychology, 8,* 296–303.

Vygotsky, L. S. (1962). *Thought and language* (E. Hanfmann & G. Vakar, Eds. & Trans.). Cambridge, MA: MIT Press.

Wechsler, D. (1997). *Manual for the Wechsler Adult Intelligence Test—Third Edition (WAIS-III).* San Antonio, TX: Psychological Corporation.

Welsh, M. C., & Pennington, B. F. (1988). Assessing frontal lobe functioning in children: Views from developmental psychology. *Developmental Neuropsychology, 4,* 199–230.

Wilding, J. (2005). Is attention impaired in ADHD? *British Journal of Developmental Psychology, 23,* 487–505.

Willcutt, E. G., Doyle, A. E., Nigg, J. T., Faraone, S. V., & Pennington, B. F. (2005). Validity of the executive function theory of attention-deficit/hyperactivity disorder: A meta-analytic review. *Biological Psychiatry, 57,* 1336–1346.

Wilson, B. A., Alderman, N., Burgess, P. W., Emslie, H., & Evans, J. J. (1996). *Behavioral Assessment of the Dysexecutive Syndrome.* Bury St. Edmunds, UK: Thames Valley Test Company.

Wolf, L. E., & Wasserstein, J. (2001). Adult ADHD: Concluding thoughts. *Annals of the New York Academy of Sciences, 931,* 396–408.

Wood, R. L. I., & Liossi, C. (2006). The ecological validity of executive function tests in a severely brain injured sample. *Archives of Clinical Neuropsychology, 21,* 429–437.

Index

Page numbers followed by *b* indicate box; *f*, figure; and *t*, table